Arthur Schopenhauer

On Vision and Colors

An Essay

Arthur Schopenhauer

On Vision and Colors

An Essay

Translated from the German by
E. F. J. Payne

Edited, with an Introduction by
David E. Cartwright

BERG
Oxford / Providence, USA

Published in 1994 by

Berg Publishers, Inc.

Editorial offices:
221 Waterman Street, Providence, RI 02906, U.S.A.
150 Cowley Road, Oxford OX4 1JJ, UK

A CIP catalogue record for this book is available from the British Library.

Library of Congress Cataloging-in-Publication Data
A CIP catalogue record for this book is available from the Library of Congress.

ISBN 0 85496 988 8

Printed in the United Kingdom by Short Run Press, Exeter.

Est enim verum index sui et falsi.
[For the truth bears evidence for itself and for the false.]

Spinoza, *Epistulae*, 74

Contents

Acknowledgements

The support, encouragement, and assistance of a number of individuals made possible this revision of E.F.J. Payne's early translation of *On Vision and Colors* (1942). Mere words are not sufficient to discharge the debt of gratitude that I owe these individuals, but I only have words to acknowledge my debt and express my gratitude. I must thank Valerie Egret-Payne for her willingness to allow me to revise the work of her father. The encouragement of Bryan Magee, John E. Atwell, Richard Larson, Wade Dazey, and Don S. Ross aided my task, as did the patience of Elyse Cartwright and Carol Lohry Cartwright. For agreeing to accept this manuscript as part of her firm's publication program, and for her willingness to make Schopenhauer's writings available in English, I thank the president of Berg Publishers, Inc., Marion Berghahn. To Vickie Bare, whose assistance was made possible by a University of Wisconsin-Whitewater Research Grant, I extend special thanks for preparing this difficult manuscript. I also thank Jeff Howard, whose careful copyediting substantially improved this text. My intellectual life has benefitted tremendously by the labors of E. F. J. Payne, for without his work I surely would have missed the genius of Schopenhauer. And if this translation does not match the standard set by Payne's other translations of Schopenhauer, the fault is mine.

D. E. C.

Schopenhauer's *On Vision and Colors*

Editor's Introduction

Arthur Schopenhauer's *Über das Sehn und die Farben: Eine Abhandlung (On Vision and Colors: An Essay)* appeared in May 1816 through the Leipzig publishing house of Johann Friedrich Hartknoch. Its publication did not go completely unnoticed. It drew one unfavorable review, and it earned Schopenhauer favorable mention in two dictionaries.[1] Yet two years after its publication, Schopenhauer would compare the sensation created by this essay to that produced by throwing a stone into a bog – no ripples![2] *Über das Sehn und die Farben* just did not receive the kind of attention that Schopenhauer desired. It failed to win the approval of its source of inspiration, Johann Wolfgang Goethe; it failed to promote the cause of Goethe's color theory; it failed to depose Newton's views; and it failed to secure recognition as "the first true theory of colors" in the history of science.[3] And so this essay suffered the same fate as the first editions of all of Schopenhauer's books except *Parerga und Paralipomena* (1851). Schopenhauer's stance toward the lack of attention paid to his essay on color theory set the tone for his attitude when his subsequent publications were ignored: the self-serving, German learned world conspired to silence the truth through indifference, but one day the truth would be recognized and its author would receive his due.

1. An anonymous review of *On Vision and Colors* appeared in *Leipziger Literature-Zeitung*, 179 (14 July 1817): pp. 1425–28 (reprinted in *Fünftes Jahrbuch der Schopenhauer-Gesellschaft* [Heidelberg, 1916], pp. 187–92). For Schopenhauer's attitude toward this review, see his letter to Goethe, 23 June 1818, in Arthur Schopenhauer, *Gesammelte Briefe*, ed. Arthur Hübscher (Bonn, 1978), p. 35. In his letter to Charles Lock Eastlake, 1841, Schopenhauer mentions favorable reference to his theory of colors in the *Conversationslexicon* and *Pierers Real Lexicon der medicinischen Wissenschaften*; see *Gesammelte Briefe*, p. 193.

2. See Schopenhauer's letter to Goethe, 23 June 1818, *Gesammelte Briefe*, p. 35.

3. Letter to Goethe, 11 November 1815, *Gesammelte Briefe*, p. 20.

Schopenhauer was patient, but he would not remain passive. He sought to hasten truth's recognition, and in 1830 he revised his essay in Latin. It appeared as "Commentatio undecima exponens Theoriam Color Physiologicam eandemque primariam" in the third volume of *Scriptores Ophthalmologici Minores*, edited by Justus Radius.[4] Schopenhauer had hoped his Latin essay would gain a foreign readership. It did not. More than a decade passed before he again lost patience. This time he adopted a different strategy. In 1841 he wrote the following to Charles Lock Eastlake, British translator of Goethe's *Zur Farbenlehre* (*On the Theory of Colors*): "May the force of truth, Sir, enlighten Your mind, and induce You to translate also this little treatise of mine, or at least to make an extract of it for the English public! This is my most fervent desire."[5] But once again the truth lacks force, and Schopenhauer's ardent desire is not sated. No translation into English is forthcoming, not even an extract. Another decade passes, and Schopenhauer senses his mortality. Fearing that it would not be possible to publish a second edition of his essay on color theory, Schopenhauer took additions planned for that edition and included them as "*Zur Farbenlehre*" ("On the Theory of Colors")[6] in the second volume of *Parerga und Paralipomena*, the very book that would earn him a readership and enable a second edition of *Über das Sehn und die Farben* in 1854.

In the second edition of *Über das Sehn und die Farben*, the "Preface" is pure Schopenhauer. As in the prefaces to the new editions of all his books published after the success of *Parerga*, Schopenhauer writes with an indignant sense of deserved triumph over the conspiracy of silence that greeted his initial publications, with an uncompromising sense of the truth of his original views, and from the stance that additions in the new addition only augment, clarify, and further justify his original views, and that only irrelevant material was deleted. In this preface he briefly describes the relationship between this new edition and the first edition, the Latin version, and the essay in *Parerga*. He does not accept blame for the con-

4. The Latin revision of *On Vision and Colors* can be found in the first volume of Arthur Hübscher's historical-critical edition of Arthur Schopenhauer, *Sämtliche Werke*, 4th ed., 7 vols. (Mannheim, 1988).

5. Letter to Eastlake, 1814, *Gesammelte Briefe*, p. 193. Schopenhauer wrote this letter in English. Eastlake's translation, *Goethe's Theory of Colors*, appeared in 1840 (reprinted, with an introduction by Deane B. Judd [Cambridge, Mass., 1970]).

6. Curiously, the title of this essay is the same as that of Goethe's book, "*Zur Farbenlehre*."

siderable delay between editions. The fault, he tells us, lies with the German public; it took them "forty years" to recognize that they would benefit by reading his books; he has remained constant, willing now, as then, to teach Goethe's color theory to Newtonians. The spirit of honesty has not failed him, Schopenhauer asserts.

Yet Schopenhauer dangles a rather curious remark in the preface. He relates that he wrote this essay in 1815 but that it was not published before Easter 1816. He attributes the delay to Goethe. He sent the manuscript to Goethe, Schopenhauer explains, and Goethe kept the manuscript longer than anticipated by taking it with him on his tour of the Rhine. Schopenhauer then proceeds to mention the indifference that greeted the publication of *Über das Sehn und die Farben* and a subsequent case of plagiarism. It is odd, however, that Schopenhauer would mention a brief delay in the appearance of a work that was greeted by indifference, and that he mentions this in a preface published thirty-eight years after the original edition appeared. Schopenhauer fails to explain why this delay is significant. Nor does he explain the connection, if any, between this incident and the failure of the first edition to attract an audience and the case of plagiarism. The explanation, of course, is that Schopenhauer is disappointed not only by the book's original reception and by the plagiarism but also by Goethe. The spirit of honesty seems not to have counseled full disclosure of the truth, however, for Schopenhauer's disappointment with Goethe does not stem merely from Goethe's delay in returning the manuscript: it is rooted in Goethe's refusal to endorse Schopenhauer's theory of colors. To understand this, it is necessary to examine the role Goethe and Goethe's theory of colors played in the genesis of *Über das Sehn und die Farben*.[7]

Unlike Nietzsche, who first fawned over Richard Wagner and then became disillusioned about Wagner and his own earlier behavior, Schopenhauer always viewed his involvement with Goethe with considerable pride. Through the tea circles held at his mother's house in Weimar, Schopenhauer became personally acquainted with

7. For an insightful discussion of Schopenhauer's intellectual relationship to Goethe, see Arthur Hübscher's *The Philosophy of Schopenhauer in its Intellectual Context*, trans. Joachim T. Baer and David E. Cartwright (Lewiston, N.Y., 1989), pp. 86–116. Rudiger Safranski provides an interesting account of Schopenhauer and Goethe's interactions concerning their work on color theory in his *Schopenhauer and the Wild Years of Philosophy*, trans. Ewald Osers (Cambridge, Mass., 1990), pp. 177–90.

Goethe. At first Goethe ignored the young Schopenhauer. But in November 1813 Goethe approached Schopenhauer, shook his hand, and congratulated the recent doctor of philosophy for his dissertation, *Über die vierfache Wurzel des Satzes vom zureichenden Grunde (On the Fourfold Root of the Principle of Sufficient Reason)*, which Schopenhauer had sent to Goethe, with a dedication, several months earlier. Goethe's favorable disposition to the young Schopenhauer was probably due to Goethe's perception of an affinity of thought between the two men, an affinity that allowed Goethe to sense a potentially important "proselyte" for his theory of colors. Schopenhauer not only shared Goethe's deep distrust of the purely conceptual but argued in his dissertation that geometrical proofs required a visual representation, a requirement Goethe had set, in his color theory, for his optical proofs.[8] Goethe needed an intelligent proponent for his theory of colors, moreover, for his massive work, *Zur Farbenlehre*, had appeared in 1810 without the reception he desired. Goethe viewed his work on color theory more highly than his poetry, and it was this theory that gave him a sense of superiority over others, but the German public did not share his judgment. So through the winter of 1813/1814 Schopenhauer and Goethe met frequently, discussing philosophy generally and color theory specifically, and they worked through a number of Goethe's color experiments. It was Goethe who induced Schopenhauer to write *Über das Sehn und die Farben*, a task that Schopenhauer would later tell Goethe was "treated only as a matter of secondary importance [*Nebensache*]" compared to the other theories he carried around constantly in his mind.[9] It is safe to say that without Goethe's encouragement Schopenhauer would not have written a work on color theory.

Schopenhauer completed the manuscript for *Über das Sehn und die Farben* in July 1815 and sent it to Goethe. He hoped that Goethe would be its editor and help secure its publication. Even more deeply, he wished for Goethe's support for his views. To Schopenhauer's great disappointment, Goethe did none of those things. He did not even indicate that he gave Schopenhauer's manu-

8. See Hübscher, *The Philosophy of Schopenhauer*, p. 90.

9. Letter to Goethe, 11 November 1815, *Gesammelte Briefe*, p. 22. The other, more important theories that he had in mind were those that would be expressed in *The World as Will and Representation* (1819). In this letter, Schopenhauer attempted to convince Goethe of the complete truth of his theory of colors by advancing a claim that he would later make about his philosophy: "My theory is the unfolding of a single, indivisible thought."

script careful consideration. After receiving a series of letters from Schopenhauer and responding to them diplomatically, Goethe returned the manuscript to its author in January 1816.

A review of the exchange of letters is instructive. Schopenhauer is bold, self-confident about his views, demanding, but always in awe of Goethe. The letters Goethe returns are noteworthy for their restraint, good-nature, and their ultimate mastery of the situation. Although Goethe had claimed to have read the manuscript, in his letter returning the manuscript he requests that Schopenhauer provide him with a summary of his views so that he could refer to them in his work.[10] Perhaps, when he received this letter, Schopenhauer recalled his earlier laments concerning Goethe's silence about his views – his failure to receive the blessings of the "godfather" of his "small child," and his beliefs that his theory followed from Goethe's "like fruit from the tree"; Goethe's "first proselyte" had to venture forth unblessed.[11] Hence Schopenhauer replies to Goethe that he could only tolerate the treatment he received during this affair from a Kant or a Goethe.[12] Schopenhauer's unhappiness, however, does not diminish his sense of Goethe's greatness. For the rest of his life he remains a proselyte for Goethe's color theory,[13] but a proselyte of a strange stripe – one who tries to set the doctrine for his teacher. But Goethe had sensed Schopenhauer's personality almost from the beginning, for shortly after the last of their meetings in Weimer, Goethe penned the following verse with Schopenhauer in mind:

> I would like to bear the teacher's burden still longer,
> If only the pupils did not at once become teachers.[14]

The pupil outreaching the teacher. This is Schopenhauer's stance towards Goethe concerning color theory. This always seems to be Schopenhauer's posture toward his heroes. To Schopenhauer, Kant and Goethe are the greatest German minds.[15] Schopenhauer views

10. Letter to Schopenhauer, 28 January 1816, *Gesammelte Briefe*, p. 497.

11. Letter to Goethe, 11 November 1815, *Gesammelte Briefe*, pp. 19, 21, 22, 24.

12. Letter to Goethe, 7 February 1816, *Gesammelte Briefe*, p. 25.

13. Almost as if to verify this, it is Goethe's theory of colors that Schopenhauer praises in his contribution to an album published in 1849 by the city of Frankfurt in honor of the centenary of Goethe's birth. Schopenhauer's entry to the album is included in *Parerga and Paralipomena*, trans. E. F. J. Payne (Oxford, 1974) vol. 2, pp. 198–200.

14. "Lahmung," in *Goethes Gedichte*, 2. Theil (Stuttgart/Tübingen, 1815), p. 199.

15. In his contribution to the Frankfurt Goethe-Album mentioned above (note 13), Schopenhauer wrote that Goethe was, "the greatest man, [of] whom, along with

his thought standing in the same relationship to both men. Kant's philosophy becomes the basis for Schopenhauer's philosophy as Goethe's color theory becomes the ground for Schopenhauer's color theory. By employing the insights of both thinkers while correcting their errors, Schopenhauer develops his own views – theories that outstrip those of their intellectual ancestors. And if Goethe read *Über das Sehn und die Farben* carefully, his letters to Schopenhauer display incredible magnanimity. Although it is only after Goethe's death, in the second edition of *Über das Sehn und die Farben* and in the earlier essay on color theory in *Parerga und Paralipomena*, that Schopenhauer wrote openly and polemically against Goethe, substantial grounds of opposition already existed in the first edition. Certainly Schopenhauer champions Goethe's theory of colors in the first edition, complains about the shabby treatment it received from the intellectual world, and adopts Goethe's anti-Newtonian stance, but there is much there at which Goethe could have taken umbrage. Schopenhauer credits Goethe for providing "abundant data" for a theory of color but claims these data do not "furnish us with a real explanation of the essential nature of color"(p. 5).[16] Schopenhauer, of course, raises Goethe's assembled data to the august height of theory. He claims that Goethe refuted Newton in the polemical part of his *Zur Farbenlehre*, but he also states that final victory over Newton is achieved only "when a new theory takes the place of an old" (p. 6). Schopenhauer's additions and corrections provide this "new theory." Even if these remarks escaped Goethe's attention during his gloss of the manuscript, Schopenhauer's letters also say as much: "I know with perfect certainty that I have produced the first theory of color, the first in the history of science."[17] And after describing to Goethe how his position "disharmonizes" with Goethe's, he

Kant, the nation boasts." Schopenhauer often associated his neglect with that of Goethe and Kant, e.g., "The fate of my philosophy and Goethe's theory of colors proves what a mean and worthless spirit is ruling over the German republic of scholars"; "Hatred of Kant, hatred of me, hatred of truth, although all *in majorem Dei gloriam*, inspire these boarders at the table of philosophy." See, respectively, *Arthur Schopenhauer, Manuscript Remains in Four Volumes*, ed. Arthur Hübscher, trans. E. F. J. Payne (Oxford/New York/Hamburg, 1988) vol. 4, "Senilia," p. 51; and Schopenhauer, *On the Will in Nature*, trans. E. F. J. Payne (Oxford/New York/Hamburg, 1992) p. 16. The "Senilia" quote also appeared in the second edition of *On Vision and Colors* but was dropped in the third edition.

16. Page references are to this translation of *On Vision and Colors*.

17. Letter to Goethe, 11 November 1815, *Gesammelte Briefe*, p. 20.

remarks, "it is not even possible for me to imagine that your Excellence would not recognize the correctness of my theory; for the truth has spoken through me – in this small matter as in days to come it will in great ones."[18] Not only does Schopenhauer claim to triumph over Goethe, he views as a "small matter" something Goethe labored on for numerous years and deemed a major accomplishment. It is not surprising that Goethe would write to Schopenhauer, "It would be a vain effort to wish for a mutual understanding."[19]

After the publication of *Über das Sehn und die Farben*, Schopenhauer sent a copy to Goethe. In his cover letter he does not request comments, telling Goethe that he had abandoned that hope and that after their earlier exchange of letters such a request would be in vain.[20] Yet he writes that if Goethe would take the trouble of reading it, he would find the manuscript changed and improved by significant additions. According to Goethe's diary entries on May 9 and 10, 1816, he did read the manuscript.[21] And although his letter in reply to Schopenhauer was cordial, he was displeased with the essay. In reply to an inquiry from a third party requesting Goethe's opinions concerning *Über das Sehn und die Farben*, Goethe wrote, "Dr. Schopenhauer is a significant thinker whom I induced to take up my theory of colors. . . . This young man, proceeding from my perspective, has become my opponent."[22]

Schopenhauer believed his split with Goethe and himself was due to Goethe's demand of "the most unqualified agreement" (p. 7), their differing views of whether gray or white consisted of a mixture of colors, the limits Schopenhauer placed on Goethe's concept of polarity, and a disagreement concerning the origin of the color violet.[23] There is, however, a deeper ground for their intellectual break, one that is beyond personal investments in the truth of their individual theories and their differences concerning color theory *per se*. As Arthur Hübscher has argued, it is Schopenhauer's Kantian commitments

18. Letter to Goethe, 23 January 1816, *Gesammelte Briefe*, p. 23.

19. Letter to Schopenhauer, 28 January 1816, *Gesammelte Briefe*, p. 496.

20. See letter to Goethe, 4 May 1816, *Gesammelte Briefe*, p. 28.

21. See *Gesammelte Briefe*, p. 499.

22. Goethe's letter to Christoph Friedrich Ludwig Schultz, 6 July 1816, quoted in *Gesammelte Briefe*, p. 499.

23. Schopenhauer explains the three ways in which his views "disharmonize" with Goethe's in his letter to Goethe, 11 November 1815, *Gesammelte Briefe*, pp. 19–20.

and with them his assignment of light and matter to a subordinate place in his color theory that constitute their intellectual split.[24] Goethe's "realism" was not compatible with Schopenhauer's transcendental idealism. Indeed, the first chapter of this essay, "*Vom Sehn*" ("On Vision") clearly articulates Schopenhauer's idealism, and Schopenhauer later claims that readers of this essay will be led to "a more profound comprehension of the Kantian doctrine of the . . . subjective, intellectual forms of all knowledge" (p. 2) by gaining a precise knowledge of the likewise subjective nature of color. Goethe's intellectual spirit certainly could not find home ground in Schopenhauer's idealism.

In *Zur Farbenlehre*, Goethe rejected the Newtonian view that white light contained the spectrum. Skeptical both of mathematical explanations, which he viewed as obscuring our understanding of nature, and of experimental instruments, since even the prism distorts reality, Goethe viewed light and darkness as primary phenomena (*Urphänomene*), basic or simple phenomena capable of no further explanation. According to Goethe, color is produced by the interplay of the polarities of lightness and darkness and is, therefore, something shadowlike or cloudy. Schopenhauer thought that as far as he went, Goethe was correct; the problem was that he did not go far enough. Goethe's "primary phenomena" were not truly "primary," Schopenhauer argued, because there was a deeper explanation for them. Color, Schopenhauer maintains, is a physiological phenomena, something in the eye alone. He explains to Eastlake: "As my theory, [*sic*] is entirely physiological, taking color as a sensation, and with respect to the eye, it is the primary theory, and anterior to all explanations of the outward causes of that sensation, which are the physical and chemical colours."[25] Since lightness or white, darkness or black, and colors are states or modifications of the eye, sensation itself, in Schopenhauer's theory, is subjective. Light or white is the full activity of the retina, dark or black is the inactivity of the retina, while color is the qualitatively divided activity of the retina. So for Schopenhauer, "Primary phenomenon properly speaking is only the organic capacity of the retina to cause its nervous activity to separate and successively appear in two qualitatively opposite halves, sometimes equal, sometimes unequal" (p. 67).

24. See Hübscher, *The Philosophy of Schopenhauer*, p. 96.

25. Letter to Eastlake, 1841, *Gesammelte Briefe*, p. 193 (Schopenhauer's English).

Based on this understanding of the physiology of colors, Schopenhauer believed that he alone produced the first true theory of colors. Schopenhauer took considerable pride in his analysis of colors in terms of definite numerical fractions, each of which, when combined with its color complement, composes a unity (one), a unity representing white, the full activity of the retina. As he expressed it to Eastlake:

> bearing in mind the numerical fractions, (of the activity of the retina) by which I express the 6 chief colours, You contemplate the colors singly, then You find that only by this, and by no other theory upon earth, You come to understand the peculiar sensation, which every colour produces in your eye, and thereby get an insight into the very essence of every colour, and of colour in general. Likewise my theory alone gives the true sense in which the notion of complementary colours is to be taken, viz: as having no reference to light, but to the retina, and not being a redintegration [*sic*] of white light, but of the full action of the retina, which by every colour undergoes a bipartition
>
> either in yellow and violet
> ¾ ¼
> or in orange and blue
> ⅔ ⅓
> or in red and green
> ½ ½
> This is in short the great mystery.[26]

Schopenhauer's numerical fractions reveal the secret of colors: "Only through such fractions do we obtain correct information concerning the true nature of colors and their difference from one another."[27] On this basis we also discover one of the central ways in which Schopenhauer's view "disharmonizes" with Goethe's, and a point on which he thought that Newton was correct. The point involves the production of white from colors. And while Schopenhauer agreed with Newton that white can be produced by colors, his agreement is, again, on the basis of a Kantian turn, so it bears only a remote analogy to Newton's view. Instead of color being the division of a ray of light, for Schopenhauer it is the divided activity of the retina, and each color becomes for Schopenhauer comprehensible as a "definite

26. Letter to Eastlake, 1841, *Gesammelte Briefe*, p. 192 (Schopenhauer's English).
27. *On the Will in Nature*, p. 32.

portion of the retina's activity, expressed by a fraction" (p. 39). The full activity of the retina, white, as we have seen above, is produced by a color and its complement. Yet despite conceding that Newton's view contains a shred of truth, Schopenhauer discounts it by arguing that it is grounded within a mistaken theory. As if he is trying to mitigate the damage his theory could do to his relationship to Goethe, Schopenhauer argues that Goethe, although wrong, had "an otherwise correct system of facts" (p. 50). Schopenhauer even seems to suggest that Newton is the cause of Goethe's confusion. Yet, to Schopenhauer, the underlying problem of both Goethe and Newton is their realism: both men mistakenly believe that colors lie outside the subject.

With this description of the genesis of *Über das Sehn und die Farben* and the sketch of Schopenhauer's theory in mind, it is worthwhile to consider the place of this essay in Schopenhauer's *oeuvre*. The question of its location in Schopenhauer's thought becomes especially intriguing when we note that this essay has drawn far less critical commentary than his other works and is not even included in the recent German-language student edition of his writings.[28] It is not surprising, however, that *Über das Sehn und die Farben* is generally ignored by Schopenhauer's commentators and readers. What draws people to Schopenhauer is his philosophy proper and the worldly wisdom of the subsidiary essays of *Parerga und Paralipomena*. And even though Schopenhauer believed that a fundamental understanding of his philosophy required reading every line he wrote, he made an exception for the lines composing *Über das Sehn und die Farben*. This essay, he tells one of his "proselytes," Ernst Otto Lindner, is not required reading, "but it is still good to read with [his other books]."[29] Schopenhauer's ambivalent attitude toward this essay is also evident in his behavior. Near the end of his life, when he contemplated an edition of his collected works, he wrote its eventual publisher, F. A. Brockhaus, a sketch that included *Über das Sehn und die Farben* as its last entry.[30] Later he seems to have changed his mind, for he wrote in his notebook "the theory of colors goes as a separate matter" from his other writings.[31] But when he carefully reworked

28. Arthur Schopenhauer, *Zürcher Ausgabe: Werke in Zehn Bänden*, (Zürich, 1977) 10 volumes.

29. Letter to Lindner, 5 January 1852, *Gesammelte Briefe*, p. 274.

30. See letter to Brockhaus, 8 August 1858, *Gesammelte Briefe*, p. 433.

31. Schopenhauer, *Manuscript Remains*, vol. 4, "Senilia," p. 97.

his books during the last decade of his life for new editions, he did so even with the second edition of *Über das Sehn und die Farben*, thereby providing the basis of Julius Frauenstädt's third edition (1870). Still, in the final editions of his various books, where he refers his readers to supporting discussions in his other writings, *Über das Sehn und die Farben* receives scant attention. This suggests, again, that it stands apart from his other writings, even though Schopenhauer's interest in color theory spanned practically his entire philosophical career.

When the collected edition of Schopenhauer's works appeared in 1873/74, Frauenstädt, its editor, included both *Über das Sehn und die Farben* and its earlier Latin version.[32] Frauenstädt justifies their inclusion in the *Sämmtliche Werke* by arguing that Schopenhauer's theories on vision and colors were an integral part of the philosopher's system, and that excluding them would make the edition incomplete.[33] He reminds his readers, moreover, of the importance Schopenhauer ascribed to this essay in the preface to the first edition of his chief work, *Die Welt als Wille und Vorstellung (The World as Will and Representation)*. There, Frauenstädt remarks, Schopenhauer requires that his readers study both *Über die vierfache Wurzel des Satzes vom zureichenden Grunde* and *Über das Sehn und die Farben* as "introductions" to his chief work. Indeed, Schopenhauer claims that the first chapter of his essay on colors, "*Vom Sehn*" would have appeared in *Die Welt als Wille und Vorstellung* "word for word" had he not been disinclined to either quote himself or use less suitable words to say for a second time something he had already said well.[34] But Frauenstädt failed to consider the context of Schopenhauer's remarks. They were made in the preface to the first edition of Schopenhauer's chief work in 1818. At that time, "*Vom Sehn*" was significant because it contained the first statement of Schopenhauer's physiological arguments for idealism. But in 1847 Schopenhauer included an expanded statement of these arguments in section 21 of the second edition of his dissertation, *Über die vierfache Wurzel des Satzes vom zureichenden Grunde*. From that point on, "*Vom Sehn*" lost its significance. Even in the preface to the second edition of *Über das*

32. Arthur Schopenhauer, *Sämtliche Werke*, ed. Julius Frauenstädt (Leipzig, 1873/74), 6 Bde.

33. See Schopenhauer, *Sämtliche Werke* (Hübscher edition), Bd. 1, pp. 8–9.

34. Schopenhauer, *The World as Will and Representation*, trans. E. F. J. Payne (New York, 1969) vol. 1, p. xiv.

Sehn und die Farben (1854), Schopenhauer calls "*Vom Sehn*" a precursor to section 21 of his dissertation, and refers his readers to that work for a better understanding of his views.[35] And, in an almost apologetic tone, Schopenhauer writes that this essay relates to philosophy "only in minor matters," but that philosophically inclined readers would profit from it through gaining knowledge of the subjective nature of colors, which would "contribute to a more profound comprehension of the Kantian doctrine of the likewise subjective, intellectual forms of all knowledge" (p. 2). Thus, Schopenhauer claims that *Über das Sehn und die Farben* serves as an introduction to philosophy. From these remarks, it appears that Schopenhauer viewed the ultimate value of *Über das Sehn und die Farben* analogously to Plato's writings, the *Vedas*, and the *Upanishads*: One need not read them to understand his philosophy, but knowledge of these works will prepare the reader to hear what he has to say by making the reader more receptive to his idealism.[36] So *Über das Sehn und die Farben* is "good to read with" his other books, but it is not required for a fundamental understanding of his philosophy.

Even if *Über das Sehn und die Farben* is not as integral to Schopenhauer's philosophy as Frauenstädt suggests, he was absolutely correct in including it in the collection of Schopenhauer's works. Yet he is correct for reasons other than mere completeness, and the essay's value lies not simply in its ability to cultivate readers' sympathy for idealism. Although it is true that *Über das Sehn und die Farben* does not present any new and significant doctrines in Schopenhauer's philosophy, it has value in that it increases our understanding of both the method and the meaning of his philosophy. This translation provides readers of English with access to an essay written early in Schopenhauer's career, when he was developing his philosophy proper. Moreover, the first chapter, "*Vom Sehn,*" contains his first detailed account of the intellectual nature of visual perception and the means by which he viewed visual experience as constructed by the understanding. Arguments based on the tremendous discrepancy between raw sensation and our perception of an external world tend to be the most persuasive arguments that he

35. P. F. H. Lauxtermann discusses the issue of the physiological arguments in his "Five Decisive Years: Schopenhauer's Epistemology as Reflected in His Theory of Color," *Studies in History and Philosophy of Science*, vol. 18 (1987) pp. 271–91.

36. See Schopenhauer, *The World as Will and Representation*, vol. 1, p. xv, for Schopenhauer's remarks about Plato, the *Vedas*, and the *Upanishads*.

developed for transcendental idealism and his anti-realist stance. The lengthy chapter "*Von den Farben*" ("On Color") also should enrich our knowledge of how Schopenhauer constructs theory based on empirical considerations. Schopenhauer claimed that "philosophy is nothing but the correct and universal understanding of experience itself, the true interpretation of its meaning and content."[37] And though Schopenhauer would regard his theory of colors as lacking the universality demanded of philosophy, its careful study may reveal in operational terms the difference Schopenhauer saw between science and philosophy.

Lastly, as Frauenstädt argued in his preface to the third edition of *Über das Sehn und die Farben*, this essay is also a significant document for the history of optics.[38] In addition to articulating Schopenhauer's theory of colors and describing numerous color experiments that he used to substantiate his theory, we find his critique of the views of both Goethe and Newton. Moreover, Schopenhauer was quite alive to the literature on color theory of that time, and there are many references to the literature in opposition to Goethe, in support of Newton, and on the topic of color theory itself. And even if one ultimately must reject Schopenhauer's theory of colors, it remains a bold intellectual construct and attempt to explain the nature of perceived colors from an idealistic perspective.

David E. Cartwright
University of Wisconsin – Whitewater
June 1992

37. Schopenhauer, *The World as Will and Representation*, vol. 2, p. 183.

38. In 1870, previous to his edition of the *Sämtliche Werke*, Frauenstädt published the third edition of *Über das Sehn und die Farben* under separate cover (Leipzig). See Frauenstädt's "Vorrede des Herausgebers zur dritten Auflage," p. x.

Note on Citations

Schopenhauer adopted the practice of referring readers of one of his books to supplementing discussions found in his other writings. In addition to the original citations to his other books found in *Über das Sehn und die Farben*, this edition provides page references for the following English-language translations of Schopenhauer's books:

On the Basis of Morality, trans. E. F. J. Payne (Indianapolis/New York, 1965).

On the Fourfold Root of the Principle of Sufficient Reason, trans. E. F. J. Payne (La Salle, Ill., 1974).

Essay on the Freedom of the Will, trans. Konstantin Kolenda, (Indianapolis/New York, 1960).

Parerga and Paralipomena, trans. E. F. J. Payne (Oxford, 1974), 2 vols.

On the Will in Nature, trans. E. F. J. Payne (New York/Oxford, 1992).

The World as Will and Representation, trans. E. F. J. Payne (New York, 1966), 2 vols.

Preface to the Second Edition

I find myself in the unusual situation of having to improve a book, for a second edition, that I wrote forty years ago. Now, just as a man always remains the same and unaltered in his kernel and true essence, though on the surface great changes take place in his appearance, manners, writing, in his style, in the trends of his tastes, in his notions, views, insights, and knowledge, and so on, through the course of the years, so by analogy this small work of my youth has also remained fully the same, because its subject matter and contents are just as true today as they were then. I have, however, made improvements in its exterior, in its arrangement, and in its form as far as was feasible. Here it has to be remembered that the hand that improves is forty years older than the hand that wrote the original work. So it was impossible to avoid the same drawback of which I have already had to complain in the second edition of the essay *Über den Satz vom Grunde*,[1] namely, that the reader is aware of two different voices, the voices of age and of youth. This is so distinct that whoever has a keen ear is never in doubt as to which is actually speaking. But it was not possible to alter this, and really it was not my fault but was ultimately due to the fact that a revered German public requires forty years in order to find out who would profit by a bestowal of its attention.

I wrote this essay in 1815, whereupon Goethe kept the manuscript longer than I had expected by taking it on his tour, at that time, of the Rhine. In this way the final editing and printing were postponed, so that the work did not appear before Easter of 1816. - Since that time neither physiologists nor physicists have found it worthy of any consideration but, quite undisturbed by it, have abided by their own words. Therefore it is no wonder that, fifteen years later, it tempted the plagiarist (as a snapper-up of unconsidered trifles, *Winter's Tale*, p. 489) to turn it to his own use. I have discussed this in detail in *Über den Willen in der Natur*, first edition, page 19, and second edition, page 14.[2]

1. [Schopenhauer's shorthand for his dissertation, *Über den vierfache Wurzel des Satzes vom zureichenden Grunde* (*On the Fourfold Root of the Principle of Sufficient Reason*).–*Trans.*]
2. [*On the Will in Nature*, pp. 30–32.–*Trans.*]

Meanwhile, I have had forty years in which to test my theory of color in all ways and on many different occasions; yet my conviction of its perfect truth has not faltered for one moment, and the correctness of Goethe's color theory is to me also still just as evident as it was forty-one years ago when he showed me his experiments. I can, therefore, assume that the spirit of truth, which reposed in me in the more weighty and important matters, has not forsaken me in this subordinate affair. This means that it is related to the spirit of honesty and seeks honest heads. – Here, of course, it has not a very great selection, especially since it demands a devotion that pays no regard either to the needs, convictions, or inclinations of the public or to the age in which it lives. Such devotion pays honor to this spirit and is prepared to teach Goethe's color theory among Newtonians, just as it is ready to preach ascetic morality among modern Protestants, Jews, and optimists.

With this second edition I have omitted only a few subsidiary discussions from the first edition that do not have a direct bearing on the subject, while on the contrary, I have enriched it by considerable additions. Between the present and first edition of this essay, there is also my revision in Latin, which I incorporated in 1830 under the title "Theoria colorum Physiologica, eademque primaria" in the third volume of the *Scriptores ophthalmologici minores*, published by Justus Radius. This is no mere translation of the first edition but differs noticeably from it in form and presentation and is also amply enriched in subject matter. Although I have used it in connection with the present edition, it still always retains its value, especially for foreign countries. Further, in 1851 I recorded in the second volume of my *Parerga und Paralipomena* a number of additions to my theory of colors in order to rescue them from destruction, because, as I stated in that work, I entertained little hope at my advanced age of living to see a second edition of the present essay. However, fate has decreed otherwise; the public attention that has at last been directed to my works has also been extended to this small and early work, although its contents relate to philosophy only in minor matters, and, in the main, concern physiology. This, however, will not be in any way unprofitable to the reader who is concerned only with philosophy, because a more precise knowledge and firmer conviction of the wholly subjective nature of color contribute to a more profound comprehension of the Kantian doctrine of the likewise subjective, intellectual forms of all our knowledge, and so it affords a very suitable introductory course of philosophy. But such a course must be all the more welcome to us, since in these days a vulgar lack of culture is gaining the upper hand and flat heads of the shallowest kind actually have the effrontery to deny, without more ado, the *a priori* and hence subjective portion of human knowledge, the discovery and separation of which is Kant's immortal contribution. At the same time, moreover, a few chemists and physiologists quite honestly imagine that they can ascertain the inner nature of things without any transcendental philosophy, and accordingly seize hold of the most naive and ingenuous realism. Without previous investigation, they simply take the objective as positively given, and it never occurs to them to take into consideration the subjective by means of which alone the objective exists. The innocence with which these people, coming from their scalpel and crucible, tackle the problems of philosophy is really astounding. Thus we see that each exclusively pursues his professional study and is afterwards ready to join in the discussion with everyone. If only we could make it clear to such men that between them and the real nature of things stands their brain, like a wall, and that, therefore, a wide detour is necessary in order to get in some measure behind it – then they would no longer recklessly dogmatize at random on "souls," "substance," and the like – just like philosophizing cobblers.[3]

Thus the additions under discussion, which were recorded for the time being in my *Parerga*, but which were there heaped together as in a lumber yard, I have had to incorporate in the present edition at their appropriate places, because I could not leave this incomplete by referring the reader to the requisite places in that chapter of *Parerga*. Naturally, the additions that are used here will be left out of the second edition of *Parerga*.[4]

Frankfurt am Main
November 1854

3.* The entire dispute between materialists and spiritualists, which has become so noisy in the year 1855–56, is merely a proof of the incredible vulgarity and shameless ignorance to which the learned vocation has sunk as a result of studying Hegelian nonsense and neglecting Kantian philosophy.

[*Footnotes marked with an asterisk are additions made by Schopenhauer in his interleaved copy of the second edition of *Über das Sehn und die Farben* (1854). These additions were incorporated in the third edition, edited by Julius Frauenstädt (Leipzig: F.A. Brockhaus, 1870). –*Trans.*]

4. [Schopenhauer, however, did not prepare a second edition of *Parerga and Paralipomena. –Trans.*]

Introduction

The subject matter of the following essay is a new theory of color, which even at the outset differs completely from all previous theories. It is written especially for those who are intimately acquainted with Goethe's color theory. Still, it will be generally comprehensible to those who know the main points of Goethe's theory, even more so if one brings along some knowledge of color phenomena, namely, of physiological phenomena, that is, those appearances of color appertaining to the eye alone, of which the most complete statement occurs in Goethe's theory of colors, although they have been earlier described more or less correctly by Buffon,[1] Waring Darwin,[2] and Himly.[3]

Buffon has the merit of being the discoverer of this remarkable fact. Its importance, indeed, its absolute necessity for a true understanding of the nature of color, is likewise apparent from my theory. For the discovery of this, however, Goethe had opened the way through a twofold service. First, in as much as he broke the old delusion of Newton's erroneous theory, he restored freedom of thought on this subject; for, as Jean Paul correctly remarks, "each revolution sooner shows itself more readily and strongly polemical than private and friendly" (*Vorschule der Aesthetik*, bd. 3, s. 861). This service, however, will gain recognition when professors' chairs and writing desks are occupied by an entirely new generation (if only this service were recognized by its elders) that does not have to hold its honor in jeopardy by the destruction of a doctrine that it expressed not as a matter of faith but as a matter of conviction throughout its life. – Goethe's second service is that he delivered in full measure what was promised by

1. *Histoire de l'académie des Sciences*, 1743. ["Dissertation sur les couleurs accidentelles." –*Trans.*]

2. Erasmus Darwin's *Zoonomia*, also [Waring Darwin, "New Experiments on the Ocular Spectra of Light and Colours, communicated by Erasmus Darwin," –*Trans.]* in *Philosophical Translations*, vol. 76.

3. *Ophthalmologische Bibliothek*, Bd. I, St. 2 ["Einiges über die Polarität der Farben," 1803, –*Trans.*]

the title of his excellent work: data for a theory of color. They are important, complete, and significant data, rich material for a future theory of color. He has not, however, undertaken to furnish the theory itself; hence, as he himself remarks and admits on page xxxix of the introduction,[4] he has not furnished us with a real explanation of the essential nature of color, but really postulates it as a phenomenon, and merely tells us how it originates, not what it is. The physiological colors, which are the point from which *my* theory starts, he represents as a phenomenon, complete and existing by itself, without even attempting to show their relation to the physical colors, his principal theme.

If theory is not based and founded thoroughly on facts, it may well be an empty and futile chimera, and each individual fragment of experience that is true has much more value. On the other hand, all the isolated facts from a definite range of the realm of experience may be completely associated, yet they do not form a science until the knowledge of their innermost nature has united them under a common conception. This conception comprises and contains all that can be found only in those facts and to which other conceptions are subordinated. By means of these we can at once arrive at a knowledge and definition of each individual fact. Such a perfected science can be compared to a well-organized state, the ruler of which can at any moment set in motion the whole, or every major portion, and also the smallest part. Therefore the comparison between the person who possesses science, the true theory, and a fact, and the person who has acquired a knowledge that is merely empirical and unorganized, although it may be extensive, is like that between a people politically organized into a kingdom and a savage tribe. This importance of theory has its most brilliant illustration in modern chemistry, the pride of our century. Its factual bases existed long before Lavoisier in the facts that had been sporadically discovered by Johann [Jean] Rey (1630), Robert Boyle, Mayow, Hales, Black, Cavendish, and finally Priestley. But they were of little use to science until they were organized into a theory in Lavoisier's great mind. This theory is, so to speak, the soul of all modern natural science by which our epoch towers above all previous epochs.

If we (here I mean the very few) see Newton's erroneous doctrine completely refuted by Goethe, partly through the polemical portion

4. [Goethe, *Zur Farbenlehre*, –*Trans.*]

of his work, and partly through a correct description of color phenomena of every kind, which Newton's doctrine had falsified, then this victory is only complete when a new theory takes the place of the old. For that which is positive has everywhere a more powerful effect on our conviction than that which is negative. Hence what Spinoza says is as true as it is beautiful: *Sicut lux se ipsam et tenebras manifestat; sic veritas norma sui et falsi est* (*Ethics*, pt. 2., prop. 43, schol.)[5]

Far be it from me to wish to pass off Goethe's work, so carefully thought out and so meritorious in every respect, as a mere aggregate of experiences. On the contrary, it is really a systematic presentation of facts, but it stops short at this. The following sentences from his "Isolated Observations and Aphorisms on Natural Science Generally," (*Nachlass*, bd. 10, s. 150, 152) testify to the fact that he felt this not without some misgiving:

> There is a weak and frail empiricism that assumes a close identity with the subject and thereby becomes real theory. – The highest attainment would be to understand that every fact was already theory. The blue color of the sky discloses the fundamental law of chromatics. Do not let us seek for anything behind phenomena, for they themselves are the theory – If I am ultimately reconciled with the primary phenomenon, then it is only from resignation; but there is still a great difference as to whether I am resigned at the extreme limits of humanity or within the narrow boundary of my limited individuality.

I hope that the theory, which I am to present, will prove that it was not the limits of humanity. In my *Parerga* (vol. 2, p. 146)[6] I have shown how this limitation was based on the purely factual in Goethe's mind, but it is not so essential to our subject that I should have to repeat it here. Thus, a theory in the proper sense is not contained in Goethe's doctrine of color, but through such a doctrine it is certainly prepared. An effort to reach such a theory is so clearly expressed in the whole work that we can say that, just as the seventh chord urgently requires the harmonic which resolves it, so a total impression of the work urgently demands a theory. Actually, the point of connection of the whole is not given in this, the point to which everything refers, the point on which everything must always depend, and to which we must always look back from each separate thing. To

5. ["Even as light displays itself and darkness, so truth is a standard for both itself and falsity." –*Trans.*]

6. [*Parerga and Paralipomena*, vol. 2, p. 178. –*Trans.*]

complete Goethe's work in this respect, to set down *in abstracto* that supreme principle on which all the data in that work rest, and thus to furnish a theory of color in the strictest sense of the word – this indeed is what the present essay will attempt to do. In the first place, of course, this will only be in regard to color considered as a physiological phenomenon. But as a result of the description now to be given, this very consideration will turn out to be the first, and indeed the absolutely essential, half of the whole theory of color. To this first half, the second, which considers physical and chemical colors, will always be theoretically in a subordinate and dependent position, although it has a greater wealth of facts.

The theory that I am about to set down is, like every true theory, indebted to the data for its origin. But since it tries first of all to explain what color is according to its essence, it will now discharge that debt by giving prominence to all these data in their proper significance by the way in which they are related, and thus they will again be firmly substantiated. Starting from this we shall even be in a position to judge *a priori,* the correctness of Newton's and Goethe's explanations of physical colors. Yes, it will be able by itself to correct those data in individual cases. So, for example, we shall in particular come across a point where Goethe is on the whole perfectly correct, yet was in error, and where Newton is on the whole completely wrong, yet to a certain extent expresses the truth, although really more in the words than in their meaning, and even so not entirely. However, on this point my departure from Goethe is the reason why he describes me, in his correspondence with Councillor Schultz, published in 1853 by Buntzer, page 149, as an opponent of his theory of colors. This was on the occasion of the present essay, in which I appear as his theory's most determined champion; and just as I was this in my twenty-eighth year, I have remained persistently so into old age. Special evidence of this is given by my large, carefully written parchment in the album published in his honor by his hometown on the centenary of his birth. From this parchment it can be seen that I am quite alone in holding aloft the standard of his theory of colors in fearless and undaunted contradiction to all the rest of the learned world.[7] He demanded the most unqualified agreement, neither more nor less. As

7. Published in *Parerga and Paralipomena*, vol. 2, p. 165 [pp. 198–200, –*Trans.*]

I had advanced an essential step beyond him through my theory, he gave vent to his ill humor in epigrams:

> I would like to bear the teacher's burdens still longer,
> If only the pupils did not at once become teachers.

What went before also alludes to this:

> Your well-conceived point in the veins of others,
> Will forthwith wrangle with you.

In the theory of colors I had been his personal pupil, and he mentions this in the above-quoted letter.

Before I come to the real subject of this essay, namely to colors, it is necessary for me to make some preliminary remarks on vision in general. The aspect of this problem, the discussion of which is required by the object I have in view, is of course not optical and physiological, but rather that aspect, which, by its very nature, comes within the province of the theory of the cognitive faculty, and consequently wholly within the domain of general philosophy. Here such an aspect appears only as a subsidiary work and could not be treated other than in a fragmentary and imperfect manner. For it appears here merely in order that, where possible, every reader will bring to the following chapter a real conviction that colors, with which objects appear to be clothed, are entirely in the eye alone. This was taught by Descartes (*Dioptrique*, c. 1) and by many others after him. It was treated most thoroughly by Locke, but long before these two men was Sextus Empiricus (*Pyrrhoniae Hypotyposes*, l. 2, c. 7, Section 72–75), who had already explained it clearly and at length. In fact he goes so far as to prove that we do not know things according to what they may be in themselves but only according to their appearances. He explains this very neatly by a simile, namely that whoever sees a picture of Socrates without knowing Socrates himself cannot say whether it is like him. Despite all this, I do not think that I can assume forthwith a clear, correct, and certain knowledge of the thoroughly subjective nature of color. But without such knowledge some scruples would constantly crop up in the following discussion on colors that would upset and weaken the persuasiveness of what is said.

What I describe here, yet only in so far as our purpose requires, thus aphoristically and in light outline – namely, the theory of the external, empirical intuitive perception [*Anschauung*] of objects in space that is brought about by the understanding and the other forms of the intellect assisting it, on the stimulation of the sensation in the sense organs – all this, I say, has in recent years been perfected by me and has been expounded clearly, comprehensively, and completely in the second edition of my essay *Über die vierfache Wurzel des Satzes vom zureichenden Grunde,* Section 21. Therefore as regards this important subject, I refer that paragraph to my reader, who must regard what is given here merely as a precursor to it.

CHAPTER ONE

On Vision

§1
Intellectual Nature of Intuitive Perception – Distinction Between Understanding and Faculty of Reason and Between Illusion and Error – Knowledge [Erkenntniss], the Characteristic of Animal Life – Application of All that is Stated to Intuitive Perception Through the Eye

All intuitive perception [*Anschauung*] is intellectual, for without the *understanding* [*Verstand*] we could never achieve intuitive perception, observation [*Wahrnehmung*], the apprehension of *objects*. On the contrary, we would stop short at the mere sensation that might possibly have meaning in reference to the will as pain or comfort; but for the rest it would be a succession of states devoid of meaning, and nothing like knowledge. Intuitive perception, that is, knowledge of an *object*, first comes about through the *understanding* that refers every impression received by the body to its *cause*. In space, which is intuited *a priori*, the understanding shifts this cause to the point from which the effect starts and thus recognizes the cause as acting, as *actual* [*wirklich*], i.e., as a representation [*Vorstellung*] of the same kind and class as the body. But this transition from the effect to the cause is direct, vivid, and necessary, for it is a knowledge of the *pure understanding*. It is not a rational conclusion, a combination of concepts and judgments according to logical laws. Such a combination is, rather, the business of *reason* [*Vernunft*], which contributes nothing to intuitive perception, but whose object is quite a different class of representations. In this world such a class belongs solely to the human race; they are abstract, not intuitive, representations; in other words, they are *concepts*. But through these man is given his great advantages such as speech, science, and above all that reflectiveness which is possible only by surveying the whole of life in concepts, and which keeps him independent of the impression of the present moment, and thus enables him to act with premeditation, deliberation, and method. In this way his actions differ so vastly from those of the animals, and finally there is also that condition for deliberate choice between several motives in virtue of which the decisions of his will are accompanied by the most complete self-consciousness. For all this, humans are indebted to *concepts*, that is, to *reason*. As an abstract principle the law of causality is naturally a reflection, like all principles *in abstracto*, and hence an object of the faculty of reason. But the real, vivid, direct, and necessary knowledge of the law of causality precedes all reflection, as it does all experience, and is to be found in the *understanding*. By means of such knowledge the body's sensations become the starting point for the intuitive perception of a world, in that the law of causality (known to us *a priori*) is applied to the relation between the immediate object (the body) and all other objects that are merely mediate. Knowledge of the same law applied solely to and among mediate objects gives us cleverness when it attains a higher degree of keenness and precision; and this can no more be produced by abstract concepts than can intuitive perception generally. Therefore, to be rational and to be clever are two very different characteristics.

Thus intuitive perception, knowledge of objects, of an objective world, is the work of the understanding. The senses are merely the seat of an enhanced sensibility; they are parts of the body that are susceptible in a higher degree to the influence of other bodies. Moreover, each sense is open to a particular kind of influence to which the other senses are either slightly susceptible or not so at all. This specific difference of sensation of each of the five senses has its ground not in the nervous system itself, but only in the way in which this system is affected. We can therefore regard each sensation as a modification of the sense of touch, or of the ability to feel, that extends over the whole body, because the substance of the nerves (apart from the sympathetic system) is in the whole body one and the same without the slightest difference. Now when it is affected by light through the eye or sound through the ear, and receives such specifically distinct sensations, this cannot reside within the substance itself, but only in the way in which it is affected. But this depends partly on the outside agent by which it is affected (light, sound, odor), and partly on the mechanism by which it is exposed to the impression of this agent, i.e., on the organ of sense. The fact that in the ear the nerve of the labyrinth and cochlea, floating in the auditory fluid, receives the vibrations of air by means of this fluid, but that the optic nerve receives the effect of light through the aqueous humor and the crystalline lens breaking up the light in the eye, is the cause of the specific difference of the two sensations, not the nerve itself.[1] Accordingly, even the auditory nerve could see and the optic nerve hear if the external apparatus of both were to change places. – However, the modification undergone by the senses through such influence is not yet by any means an intuitive perception, but only the material which the understanding converts into such a perception. Of all the senses, that of sight is capable of the most delicate and diverse impressions from without; yet in itself it can give only sensation which first becomes intuitive perception through the application of the understanding. If anyone standing before a beautiful landscape could for a moment be deprived of all understanding, then for him nothing of the whole view would be left but the sensation of a very manifold affection of his retina, resembling the many blobs of different colors on an artist's palette. These are, so to speak, the raw material from which just a moment previously his understanding created that intuitive perception.[2] – In the first weeks of life the infant feels with all its senses; it does not intuitively perceive, does not apprehend; it therefore stares stupidly at the world. Yet it soon begins to learn the use of its understanding, to apply the law of causality that is known prior to all experience, and to combine this with the forms of all knowledge, time and space, which are likewise given *a priori*. Thus from sensation it arrives at intuitive perception, at apprehension, and it then looks at the world with shrewd, discerning, and intelligent eyes. But each object operates differently on all five senses, and yet these effects lead back to one and the same cause, which, precisely in this way, presents itself as object. Therefore the infant learning intuitive perception compares the different kinds of impressions it receives from the same object. It touches what it sees and examines what it touches; according to the sound, it proceeds to its cause, bringing to aid smell and taste; finally, it also takes into account distance and illumination by its eyes. It becomes acquainted with the effect of light and shade, and in the end, after much effort, it also becomes familiar with perspective, knowledge of which is brought about through the union of the laws of space with the law of causality. These two reside *a priori* in

1. Cabanis, *Des rapports du physique et du moral* [*de l'homme*, –*Trans.*]: *Mémoire*, III, Section 5.

2. This concerns the pages that Herr Prof. Rosas of Vienna appropriated. I have mentioned this and his other plagiaries in *On the Will in Nature*, 2nd ed., p. 14f. ["Physiology and Pathology," pp. 30–32, –*Trans.*]

consciousness and require only application. Now here we must take into account even the changes undergone partly by the inner conformation of the eyes and partly by the mutual position of the two eyes when they see at different distances. For the understanding, all these combinations are already made by the infant, but for the faculty of reason, that is, *in abstracto*, only by the optician. Thus the infant elaborates the manifold data of sensibility into *intuitive perception* in accordance with the laws of the *understanding* that are known *a priori*. With that perception, the world first of all exists as an object. Much later it learns to use *reason*; it then begins to understand speech, to talk, and to *think* in the real sense of the word.

What is said here about intuitive perception will be even more illuminating from a more detailed consideration of the matter. The very first requirement for the acquisition of intuitive perception is that objects stand upright, even though their impression is upside down. That is to say, because the rays of light coming from a body cross when they pass through the pupil, the impression they make on the nervous substance of the retina, which has been erroneously called its image, comes through in an inverted order. Thus light coming from the bottom arrives at the top, that from the top at the bottom, that from the right arrives on the left, and vice versa. Now if, as was assumed, an actual image on the retina were the object of intuitive perception that was then bought about in some way by a soul sitting at the back of the brain, then we would see the object inverted, as actually happens in every camera that receives through a mere hole the light from external objects. Here it is not so; instead intuitive perception is brought about by the fact that the understanding instantly refers the impression felt on the retina to its cause, which then precisely in this way presents itself as an object in space, which is its accompanying form of intuition. By thus going from the effect back to the cause, the understanding follows the direction inevitably followed by the sensation of the rays of light. Thus everything is back again in its right place, for what was in the sensation at the bottom now appears in the object at the top. – The second requirement for the acquisition of intuitive perception is that, although the infant sees with two eyes, each of which receives a so-called image of the object, and indeed in such a way that the direction from the same point to each eye is different, it nevertheless learns to see only *one* object. This occurs simply by virtue of the original knowledge of the law of causality by which the effect of a point of light is recognized as causally originating from *one* point and object, although it impinges on each eye from a different direction. The two lines from that point through the pupils onto each retina are called the optical axes, and their angle at that point is the optical angle. If, when observing an object, each eyeball has the same position with respect to its own orbit, as is the case in the normal state, then in each of the two eyes the optical axis will rest on *mutually corresponding, homonymous* spots of the retina. Here it is not the outer side of one retina that corresponds to that of the other; rather, the right side of the left retina corresponds to the right side of the right, and so on. With this regular position of the eyes in their orbits, which is maintained in all the natural movements of the eyes, we now become empirically acquainted with the spots that exactly correspond to one another on the two retinas, and henceforth refer the affections originating on these analogous spots always to one and the same object as their cause. Therefore, although we see with two eyes and receive double impressions, we cognize and perceive everything only singly. That which is *doubly felt though the senses* is only *singly perceived intuitively*, simply because intuitive perception is intellectual and not merely sensuous. – But that it is the conformity of the affected spots of each retina, to which we agree in the case of every *influence of the understanding*, can be proven from the fact that, while the optical axes are directed to a more distant object, closing the optical angle, an object standing nearer to us appears double because the light coming from it through the pupils to the retinas now impinges on two spots that are not analogous. Conversely, for the same reason, the more distant object is seen double if we direct our eyes to the nearer object and close the optical angle accordingly. In the second edition of my essay *On the Fourfold Root*, there is a plate that gives a graphic description of the matter and is very useful for a thorough comprehension of it.[3] In Robert Smith's *Optics*, Cambridge, 1738, will be found a detailed description, illustrated with many figures, of the different positions of the optical axes and of the phenomena produced.

This relation between the optical axes and the object is fundamentally no different from the case in which the impression, made on each of the ten fingers in contact with an object differs in accordance with the position of each finger, but is nevertheless perceived and recognized as resulting from *one* object. Knowledge of an object

3. [*On the Fourfold Root of the Principle of Sufficient Reason*, p. 89. –*Trans.*]

never results from the mere impression, but always only from the application of the law of causality, and consequently of the understanding. – Incidentally, it is thus quite absurd to represent knowledge of the law of causality as springing first from experience, for example, experience of the resistance that objects offer to our pressure. For the law of causality is the sole form of the understanding and the precondition of the possibility of any objective perception. It is also the preliminary condition of our perception of those objects which again must first be the motive of our acting on them. And if the understanding did not already possess the law of causality and bring it ready-made to the sensation, how then could that motive arise from the mere feeling of a pressure in the hands which is absolutely nothing like that motive? (On causality between the will and bodily action, see *Die Welt als Wille und Vorstellung*, 3rd ed., 2, p. 41–44, and *Über den vierfache Wurzel des Satzes Grunde*, 2nd ed., p. 4).[4] If the English and French are still burdened with such buffoonery, we can put this down to their artless innocence, since the Kantian philosophy has not yet sunk into them and they are therefore still involved in the inadequate empiricism of Locke and Condillac. But if today German philosophasters presume to pass off time, space, causality as knowledge drawn from experience, and offer for sale absurdities that have been completely set aside and exploded for seventy years, and at which even their grandfathers shrugged their shoulders (in the meantime there lurk behind such marketing certain designs that I have exposed in the preface to the second edition of *Über den Willen in der Natur*), they deserve to be confronted with the *Xenien* of Goethe and Schiller:

> Poor empirical devil! you do not even know
> The dullness in you; it is alas so *a priori* dull.

In particular I advise everyone unfortunate enough to possess a copy of the third edition of Ernst Reinhold's *System der Metaphysik*, 1854, to write this verse on the title page. – Because the *a priori* nature of the law of causality is so obvious, even Goethe speaks of "the *most inborn conception*, the most necessary concept of cause and effect"; and he was not otherwise concerned with investigations of this sort, and merely followed in his own feelings. (Cf. *Ueber Naturwissenschaft im*

4. [See *The World as Will and Representation*, vol. 2. chap. 4, and *On the Fourfold Root*, p. 114. –*Trans.*]

allgemeinen in the tenth volume of his posthumous works.) However, I return to our theory of empirical intuitive perception.

After intuitive perception has long been acquired, there can occur a very remarkable situation that furnishes, as it were, a proof of all that has been said. Thus after we have practiced at every moment for many years the business, learned in childhood, of elaborating and arranging the data of sensibility in accordance with the laws of the understanding, such data can become confused through a change in the position of our organs of sense. Two cases in which this occurs are well known, namely, shifting the eyes from their regular natural position as in looking cross-eyed, and crossing the middle and index fingers of one hand. In these situations we see and touch *one* object as *double*. As always, the understanding correctly goes to work, but it receives nothing but false data; for the rays of light proceeding from a single point to the two eyes no longer impinge on the two retinas at mutually corresponding spots, and the outer sides of the two fingers touch the opposite surfaces of the same ball, which could never happen with the natural position of the fingers. The result is double sight and double touch as a false appearance that cannot possibly be removed, since the understanding does not at once abandon the application so laboriously acquired but continues to assume the position of the sense organs that prevailed until this time. – But an even more striking proof of our theory, because it is more unusual, is furnished by the opposite case in which we see *two* objects as *one*. This occurs when each of the objects is seen with a different eye. Let us arrange two similar cardboard tubes parallel to each other so that the distance between them is equal to that between the eyes. Fix a coin vertically in the object end of each tube. If we now look through the tubes with both eyes, we will see only *one* tube and *one* coin, because the optical axes cannot close the optical angle that would be suitable to this distance. On the contrary, the axes remain quite parallel, since each follows its tube, whereby the corresponding spots of each retina are now affected by a different coin. The understanding then attributes this double impression to one and the same object and therefore apprehends only one object where there are nevertheless two. – The recently invented stereoscope also depends on this phenomenon. For this purpose two daguerreotypes are taken of the same object, yet from a slightly different position, which corresponds to the parallax from one eye to the other. The daguerreotypes are now placed side by side at the very obtuse angle suitable to this parallax, and are then viewed through the binocular tube. The results are (1) that the symmetrically corresponding spots of the two retinas are affected by the same points of the two pictures; and (2) that each of the two eyes sees *that* part of the photographed body that, because of the parallax, remains hidden from the other eye. In this way we get not only the two pictures merging into one in the intuitive apprehension of the understanding, but also, in consequence of the second circumstance, the perfect manifestation of a solid body. A mere painting, even one produced by the greatest art and skill, never produces such a deception, because it always shows us its objects only as a one-eyed person would see them. I do not know how a proof of the intellectual nature of intuitive perception could be more striking. Without a knowledge of this, we will never understand the stereoscope but will make futile attempts with purely physiological explanations.

We now see that all these illusions result from the fact that the data, to which the understanding learned in earliest infancy to apply its laws and has throughout life become accustomed, are shifted in that they are placed in a position different from that which they occupy in the natural course of things. But at the same time, this consideration offers so clear a view of the difference between understanding and reason that I cannot refrain from drawing attention to it. Thus it is true that for reason such an illusion can be removed, but it cannot be destroyed for the understanding, which, because it is pure understanding, is nonrational. What I mean is that with such an intentionally arranged illusion we *know* quite well *in abstracto*, and hence for the *faculty of reason*, that for example, only *one* object exists, although we see and touch two respectively with crossed eyes and fingers; or that two exist, although we see only *one*. But in spite of this abstract knowledge, the illusion itself still persists, fixed and unmoved; for understanding and sensibility are inaccessible to the principles of reason, in other words, they are entirely void of reason. From this we see what *illusion* [*Schein*] and *error* [*Irrtum*] really are; the former is deception of the understanding and the latter that of *reason*; the former is opposed to *reality*, the latter to *truth*. Illusion [*Schein*] invariably results from the fact that to the always regular and unalterable apprehension of the *understanding* is attributed a state of the organs of sense that is unusual, in other words, different from the one to which it has learned to apply its functions. Or again, illusion arises from the fact that an effect, which the senses receive normally every day and hour from one and the same cause, is for once produced by an entirely different cause. This happens, for instance, when we mistake a painting for a relievo; or a stick plunged into water appears broken; or a concave mirror shows an object as floating in front of it, a convex one showing it as behind; or the moon appears much larger on the horizon than at its zenith. This is due not to refraction but simply to the direct assessment of size that is carried out by the understanding according to distance, and this again, as with terrestrial objects, according to atmospheric perspective, that is, to cloudiness through vapor and smoke. – *Error* on the other hand, is a *judgment of reason*, which does *not* stand to that which is required by the particular form of the principle of sufficient reason unique to the faculty of reason;[5] thus error is an actual, yet false, judgment, a groundless assumption *in abstracto*. Illusion [*Schein*] can give rise to error; for example, in the case already quoted, the judgment "here are two balls," which stands to nothing in the aforesaid relation and thus has no ground. On the other hand, the judgment "I feel an effect similar to that of two balls" is true, for it stands to the felt affection in the above-mentioned relation. Error can be effaced precisely through a judgment that is true and has the illusion as its ground, in other words, through a statement of the illusion as such. Illusion, however, cannot be eliminated; for instance, the moon does not become smaller because of the abstract knowledge of the faculty of reason that an estimation according to atmospheric perspective and the greater density of smoke and vapor in a horizontal direction make it larger. Nevertheless the illusion may gradually disappear when its cause is permanent and the unusual becomes, by the action of the illusion, the usual. If, for example, a man crosses his eyes, his understanding tries to correct its apprehension and to produce, through a correct grasp of the external cause, an agreement between perceptions obtained in different ways, as between seeing and touching. It then does afresh what it did in the child, and now becomes acquainted with the spots on each retina which, with the new position of the eyes, are now affected by the ray of light coming from *one* point. Therefore, humans permanently cross-eyed still see everything singly. If through an accident, such as paralysis of the eye muscles, a man is *suddenly* forced into a constant state of cross-eyedness, then at the outset he sees everything double.

5. [Schopenhauer's reference here is to the principle of sufficient reason of knowing, which assers that judgments must have as a ground or reason something other than themselves to be true. See *On the Fourfold Root of the Principle of Sufficient Reason*, p. 156. –*Trans.*]

As evidence of this, there is the case reported by Cheselden (*Anatomy*, 3rd ed., p. 324) where a man received a blow on the head, and his eyes assumed a permanently distorted position. He now saw everything double, but after some time he again had single vision, although his eyes remained out of parallel. A similar case is found in the *Ophthalmologische Bibliothek* (vol. 3, pt. 3, p. 164). If the patient described there had not made a quick recovery, he would have been permanently cross-eyed, but in the end would no longer have seen double. Yet another case of this kind is related by Home in his lecture in the *Philosophical Transactions* for 1797. – Likewise a man who always kept his fingers crossed would in the end cease to have a double touch. But so long as a man looks cross-eyed each day at a different optical angle, he will see everything double. – For the rest, it may always be as Buffon states (*Histoire de l'académie des sciences*, 1743) that those with a very pronounced and inward cross-eyedness do not see at all with the distorted eye; but this will not apply to all cases of cross-eyedness.

Now as there is no intuitive perception without understanding, all animals undoubtedly have this faculty. In fact understanding distinguishes animals from plants, just as reason distinguishes human beings from animals. For *knowledge* [*Erkennen*] is the really outstanding *characteristic of animals*, and this positively calls for understanding. Many different attempts have been made to establish a mark of difference between animals and plants, but nothing entirely satisfactory has ever been found. The most felicitous expression was always *motus spontaneus in victu sumendo*.[6] But this is only a phenomenon established by knowledge and thus subordinate to it. For a truly arbitrary and spontaneous movement, not resulting from mechanical, chemical, or physiological causes, takes place entirely in accordance with a *known object* that becomes the *motive* of that movement. Even when the polyp, that animal standing nearest to the plant, seizes its prey with its tentacles and directs it to its mouth, it has seen and perceived it (although as yet without separate eyes); and without understanding it would never have reached even this intuitive perception. The intuitively perceived object is the motive of the polyp's movement. – I would therefore lay down the following distinction between inorganic bodies, plants, and animals. An *inorganic body* is one whose every movement happens due to an external cause. The cause is equal to the effect, so that from the cause the effect can be measured and

6. ["Spontaneous movement in the taking of food." –*Trans.*]

calculated. The effect also produces in the cause an absolutely equal countereffect. A *plant* is that which has movements, the causes of which are by no means equal according to the degree of the effects. These causes afford no measure or standard for the effects, nor do they undergo an equal countereffect; such causes are called *stimuli.* Not only the movements of sensitive plants and of the *Hedysarum gyrans*, but all assimilation, growth, tendency to light, etc., in plants are movement on stimuli. Finally, an *animal* is that which has movements ensuing not directly and simply in accordance with the law of causality, but in accordance with that of motivation; and motivation is causality that has passed through knowledge and has this as its intermediary. Consequently, an animal is simply that which knows, and *knowledge is the real and proper characteristic of animals.* It must not be urged that knowledge cannot furnish us with any characteristic feature because, finding ourselves outside the being to be judged, we cannot say whether or not it knows. This we certainly can do, for we can judge whether the thing on which its movements ensue acted on it as *stimulus* or as *motive*; of this we can never be left in any doubt. For although stimuli differ from causes in the way I have mentioned, they nevertheless have in common with them the fact that, in order to operate, they always need contact, frequently even intussusception, but always a certain duration and intensity of impression. On the other hand, the object operating as a motive needs only to be perceived, it matters not for how long, at what distance, or how distinctly, so long as it is actually perceived. It goes without saying that in many respects the animal is at the same time plant and even inorganic body. This very important distinction of the three stages of causality, which is presented here only briefly and aphoristically, is found discussed specifically and in more detail in *Die beiden Grundprobleme der Ethik,* [*The Two Fundamental Problems of Ethics*], the first-prize essay in Chapter 3, and also in the second edition of the essay *Über die vierfache Wurzel des Satzes vom zureichenden Grunde*, Section 20.

Finally, I now come to that which contains a reference to what has been so far said about our theme proper, namely *colors*, and I thus proceed to a very special and subordinate part of the intuitive perception of the corporeal world. For just as the intellectual share of intuitive perception, previously considered, is really the function of the brain, namely of a considerable mass of nerves weighing from three to five pounds, so in the following chapter I have to consider simply the function of the fine nervous membrane at the back of the eye- ball, namely the *retina*. I will show that the retina's specially modified activity is color, which, perhaps as something additional and superfluous, clothes intuitively perceived bodies. Thus intuitive perception, that is, apprehension of an objective corporeal world filling space with its three dimensions, originates through the understanding, for the understanding, and in the understanding, as was previously pointed out in general but discussed in more detail in Section 21 of the essay *On the Fourfold Root*. Like space and time, the forms underlying the understanding, the understanding is a function of the brain. The senses are merely the points of departure for this intuitive perception of the world. Their modifications are therefore given prior to all intuitive perception; as mere sensations they are the data from which the intuitive perception of knowledge first comes about in the understanding. Foremost of these is the impression of light on the eye, and then color as a modification of that impression. These then are the affection of the eye, are the effect itself, which exists even without any relation to a cause. The newborn infant has the sensation of light and color before it intuitively perceives and knows the luminous or colored object as such. Not even any cross-eyedness alters the color. If the understanding converts the sensation into intuitive perception, then naturally this effect is also related and assigned to its cause, and to the body producing the effect; light or color are attributed as qualities, that is to say, as modes of operation. Yet the body is recognized only as that which produces this effect. "The body is red" means that it produces the effect of color in the eye. To be [*sein*] is generally synonymous with to act [*wirken*]; accordingly, even in German, everything that *is*, is very strikingly and with unconscious profundity called *actual* [*wirklich*], that is, acting [*wirkend*]. – By our apprehension of color as something inherent in a body, the immediate perception of it that precedes this is by no means changed. It is and remains an affection of the eye; the object is intuitively perceived merely as the cause of that affection. But color itself is only the effect [*Wirkung*]; it is the state produced in the eye, and as such is independent of the object, which exists only for the understanding; for all intuitive perception is intellectual.

CHAPTER TWO

On Colors

§2

Full Activity of the Retina

It follows from our previous observations that brightness, darkness, and color, taken in the strictest sense, are immediately felt conditions, modifications, of the eye. A well-founded consideration of color must proceed from this conception and must therefore begin by investigating color as a physiological phenomenon. For in order to go to work properly and deliberately, before we undertake the discovery of the cause of a given effect, we must become thoroughly acquainted with this effect, because only from the effect can we gather data for the discovery of the cause, and only the effect furnishes us with the direction and clue to this. Newton's fundamental mistake was simply this. Without obtaining some accurate knowledge of the effect according to its inner reference and relation, he was in too much of a hurry to go in search of the cause. Yet this same mistake is common to all theories of color from the oldest to the latest of Goethe. All speak about what modifications either the surface of a body or light must undergo, whether through analysis into its component parts or through cloudiness or other obscuration, in order to exhibit color, in other words, to stimulate in our eye that thoroughly specific sensation that cannot be described, but that can be demonstrated only through the senses. Instead of this, it is obvious that the correct way is first to turn our attention to the sensation itself, in order to explore whether we might not elicit from its nature and regular conformity that of which it consists in and by itself, hence what it is physiologically. Obviously such an accurate knowledge of the effect, which is the point in question when speaking of colors, will furnish us with data for finding the cause, in other words, for discovering the external stimulus that excites such a sensation. To begin with, for every possible *modification* of an effect, it must be possible to demonstrate a *modifiability* of its cause exactly corresponding to that effect. Further, where the modifications of the effect are not separated from one another by sharp lines of demarcation, such lines should not be drawn in the cause, but here, too, the same gradualness of the transitions must take place. Finally, where the effect exhibits contrasts, that is, admits of a complete reversal of its character, then the conditions for this must also lie in the nature of the cause according to Aristotle's rule: τῶν γὰρ ἐναντίων τὰ ἐναντία αἴτια (*nam contrariorum contrariae sunt causae. De Generatione et Corruptione*, bk. 2, cap. 10.).[1] In accordance with all of this, we shall find that my theory, which considers color only in itself, that is, as a given specific sensation in the eye, already furnishes us data *a priori* for judging the theories of Newton and Goethe concerning the objective aspect of color, that is, on the external causes that stimulate such a sensation in the eye. It will then be seen that everything speaks in favor of Goethe's theory and against Newton's. – Thus only after the consideration of color as such, that is, as a specific sensation in the eye, can we embark on a wholly different consideration; namely, the consideration of the external causes of those special modifications of the sensation caused by light, that is, the consideration of those colors that Goethe has quite correctly divided into physical and chemical.

It is the undoubted teaching of physiology that all sensibility is never pure passivity, but reaction to a received stimulus. This teaching has already been expressed by Aristotle in special reference to the eye, and particularly in so far as the eye sees colors. He says: Οὐ μόνον πάσχει, ἀλλὰ καὶ ἀντιποιεῖ τὸ τῶν χρωμάτων αἰσθητήριον (*non modo patitur sensorium, quo natura colorum percipitur, sed etiam vicissim agit. De Somniis*, chap. 2.)[2] – Among others we find a very convincing discussion of the matter in Darwin's *Zoonomia*, page 19, et seq. – I will call that reaction to external stimulus, peculiar to the eye in general, its *activity*, and in fact more specifically, the activity of the *retina*. The retina is undoubtedly the seat of that which, during vision, consists in mere sensation. What by itself provokes this activity, immediately and primarily, is *light*. The eye receiving the full impression of light manifests the *full activity of the retina*. With the absence of light, i.e., with *darkness*, *inactivity* of the retina takes place.

Bodies that under the influence of light react on the eye just like light itself are *shining* or *mirrors*.

Those bodies, however, are *white*, and when exposed to the influence of light do not react on the eye quite like light itself but with a

1. ["For contrary effects demand contraries as their causes"; p. 336a, –*Trans.*]
2. ["The organ that perceives color is not only affected by its object, but also reacts upon it"; p. 460a, –*Trans.*]

small difference, namely with a certain mellowing and equable diffusion. If we do not intend to pass from the appearance in the eye to its cause, then we could not define such mellowing more closely than that it is the absence of brightness and the radiant quality of light. Just as we distinguish radiant heat from diffused heat, so we might call white diffused light. But if we wish to express the effect through the cause, then Goethe's explanation of white appearing in the physical way, that it is complete cloudiness, is thoroughly appropriate and correct. Bodies that do not react at all under the influence of light are *black*.

Radiance is not taken into account in this entire discussion, because it is something that does not concern our subject. White is regarded as light that reacts, and therefore the effect on the eye of both (namely of light and of white) is regarded as essentially the same. We therefore say that under the influence of light or white, the *retina is in full activity*; with the absence of both of these, in other words, with darkness or blackness, *inactivity* of the retina occurs.

§3
Intensively Graduated Activity of the Retina

The influence of light and white on the retina and the retina's ensuing activity have degrees in which, by constant and steady transition, light comes near to darkness and white to shadow. In the former case they are called half or partial shadows, and in the latter gray. We therefore obtain the two following series of gradations of the retina's activity, which form essentially only *one* series, and which appear separate merely through the minor circumstance of the immediate or mediate influence of the stimulus:

Light; Half Shade; Darkness.
White; Gray; Black.

The degrees of lesser activity of the retina (half shade and gray) indicate only a partial intensity of activity. I therefore call the possibility of these degrees in general the *intensive divisibility of the retina's activity*.

§4
Extensively Graduated Activity of the Retina

Just as we found the activity of the retina intensively divisible, the same also can be found of this activity concerning its extensive divisibility because this activity is inherent in an extended organ. In this way, an *extensive divisibility of the activity of the retina* is acknowledged.

The existence of this divisibility already follows from the fact that the eye can receive many different impressions simultaneously, and hence side by side. It is, however, brought into special prominence by the experiment described by Goethe (*Zur Farbenlehre*, vol. 1, pp. 9 and 13); after having looked for a short time at a black cross on a white background and then to a gray or dim surface, the reverse phenomenon is produced in the eye, namely a white cross on a black background. The experiment can be made on the crossbar of a window at any time. The explanation of this phenomenon is as follows: on those spots of the retina that were affected by the white background, the retina's activity is so exhausted by this stimulus that, directly after this, it can no longer be perceptibly excited by the lesser stimulus of the gray surface. This surface, on the other hand, acts with its whole force on the remaining spots, previously affected by the black cross and resting during this inactivity, and here, accordingly, it produces an intensive degree of the retina's full activity. Therefore the reversal of the phenomenon here is really only apparent; at any rate it is not spontaneous, as one might be inclined to believe, i.e., it is not a real action that the previously rested part produced *by its own accord*. For if, as Goethe also mentions (*Zur Farbenlehre*, vol. I, part 1, Section 20), after the received impression, we close the eye (here, however, our eyes must be covered with our hand), or look into complete darkness, the phenomenon is not reversed, but rather the received impression simply lasts for some time. This fact would not be reconcilable with that assumption. If, however, we neglect to cover the eyes with the hand, then the light that penetrates the eyelids will produce the above mentioned effect of a gray surface, and the phenomenon will then of course be reversed. That this is the consequence of the penetrating light just mentioned follows from the fact that, as soon as we cover the eyes with our hand, the reversed phenomenon ceases at once. Franklin also conducted this experiment, and Goethe repeats the report on it in the historical portion of his *Zur Farbenlehre*. It is necessary to be quite clear on this, so that we shall know the essential difference between this phenomenon and the one now to be discussed.

§5
Qualitatively Graduated Activity of the Retina

The intensive and extensive divisibility of the retina's activity, which have been described so far, and which are subject to no doubt, can be classified under the general conception of a *quantitative divisibility of the activity of the retina.* Now it is my intention to show that yet a third can take place, a *qualitative* division of this activity, that is *toto genere* different from the other two, and that this is actually accomplished as soon as any *color* is presented, in whatever way it may be, to the eye. The phenomenon mentioned at the end of the preceding paragraph offers us a convenient point of transition to this discussion. I will once more bring it to our notice.

Here, however, I must first make it clear to the reader that to understand the real kernel of my following theory of colors, observation is indispensable, and the reader must carry out the experiments to be mentioned. Fortunately this is extremely easy. We require nothing more than a few pieces of brightly colored paper or silk ribbon in the colors we are going to consider. We cut them into disks, the form assumed here, or indeed in any other form, and make them each a few square inches. We fasten them lightly on a gray or white door, and then, after looking steadily at them for some thirty seconds, we quickly pull them away, at the same time keeping our eye on the place they occupied. Now instead of the original color, we see a totally different color in the same figure. This cannot fail to occur. If we do not perceive it at once, this is due to a lack of the required attention and habit of concentration. The experiment demands the greatest energy if we stick the pieces of vividly colored silk on the window pane where we see them penetrated by light. – But without this observation, we shall not really know the result of our report, and will just drag around in mere words.

Therefore, let us first look at a white disk on a black background for twenty or thirty seconds, and then look at a dim or light gray surface; a black disk on a bright background will then be revealed to the eye. This is still entirely the phenomenon of *extensive* divisibility of the retina's activity. On that spot of the retina that was affected by the white disk, the visual power is exhausted for the time being, and thus its complete inactivity takes place under a weaker stimulus. This can be compared to a drop of sulfuric ether evaporating on the hand and extracting the heat from that spot until the heat is gradually restored.

Now let us put a *yellow* disk in place of the white. If we now look at the gray surface, then instead of the black disk that indicated complete inactivity of this spot of the retina, we shall see a *violet* disk. This is what Goethe appropriately calls the physiological color spectrum,[1] just as he has described all the relevant facts with great accuracy and exhaustive thoroughness, but he has not gone beyond this. But for the present we are concerned with the explanation of the event, hence with the physiological process that goes on here, and it becomes all the more serious, in my opinion, because only from its correct explanation is a true comprehension of the real nature of color generally possible; but such an explanation clearly emerges, if we apply our eyes and heads at the same time. That is to say, from the intuitive perception of the aforesaid phenomenon, and from the careful comparison of what follows upon seeing a white disk with what follows from seeing a yellow one, the following explanation of the proceeding phenomenon, at first not capable of proof, yet requiring one, results as just the immediate judgment of the phenomenon itself, because it is simply the correct expression of the same. For here we have reached the point where the sensuous impression has done its part and can give nothing more, and where it is the turn of the faculty of judgment to understand and express what is empirically given. However, the correctness of this explanation will be more and more apparent from our further discussion, which will follow this phenomenon through its various phases, and it will finally obtain full corroboration through the proof of the matter to be given in Chapter 10.

With the appearance of the *yellow* disk in the eye, the *full* activity of the retina was not stimulated and more or less exhausted, as it was previously by the *white* disk. Rather, the yellow disk was able to develop only a part of the activity of the retina, leaving behind the other part, so that the activity of the retina has now been *qualitatively divided* and has separated into two halves, one of which manifested itself as a *yellow* disk; the other lagged behind and now of its own accord follows as a *violet* spectrum without any new external stimulus. In the case of this phenomenon, both the yellow disk and the violet spectrum, as the separate qualitative halves of the retina's full activity, are equal to this full activity when taken together. Therefore, *in this sense* I call each the *complement* of the other. Furthermore, as the

1. [Schopenhauer uses the word "spectrum (*Spektrum*)" in the same sense as Goethe, as "after-image." –*Trans.*]

impression of yellow comes much nearer to that of full light or white than does the impression of violet, we must at once add a second assumption, namely that the *qualitative halves*, in which the retina's activity was here divided, are *not equal* to one another, but rather the yellow color is a much greater qualitative portion of this activity than is its complement, the violet color. We should observe, however, that the *unessential* light and dark, which is the mixture of the color with white or black and which has still to be specially considered, is not meant here and has nothing to do with this case. Every color,in fact, has a point of maximum purity and freedom from all white and black, and on Runge's ingeniously contrived *color sphere* this point is represented by the equator, lying equidistant from the white and black poles. On this equator all the colors are laid out with quite imperceptible transitions from the one to the other, so that red, for instance, on one side very gradually passes into orange, orange into yellow, yellow into green, green into blue, and blue into violet; violet again comes back to red. All these colors, however, appear in full energy only at the equator, and lose more and more of this energy toward the black pole through darkening and toward the white pole through fading. Therefore, at the point of its maximum energy, as represented by the equator, each color has an intrinsic and essential approximation to white, or a resemblance to the impression of full light; and, on the other hand, an obscure haziness corresponding inversely to this, hence an approximation to darkness. Through this degree of brightness or darkness, peculiar and essential to each color, they are accordingly different from each other, apart from their other differences, because one is nearer to white, another nearer to black; and this difference is obvious. That intrinsic brightness essential to color is very different from all brightness given to it by incidental admixture, because the color retains it in the state of its greatest energy, but the white that is contingent and mixed with it diminishes it. Thus, for example, violet is essentially the most somber and ineffective of all colors; yellow, on the other hand, is essentially the brightest and most cheerful. Now violet can of course become very bright through an admixture of white, but it does not thereby obtain any greater energy; on the contrary, it loses even more of its own characteristic energy and is converted into a pale, subdued lilac or pale violet, similar to a light gray, which cannot in any way be compared with the energy of blue. Conversely, by an admixture of black, we can impart to all colors, and even to the essentially brightest, any desired degree of darkness. But such enforced darkening also directly diminishes their energy, as for example, when we get brown from yellow. In the effectiveness of the colors as such, thus in their energy, it is possible to know whether they are pure and free of all black or white foreign to their nature. By its intrinsic, essential brightness, yellow announces itself as an incomparably greater qualitative part of the eye's activity than its complement, violet, the most somber.

Now let the yellow disk previously used as an example become *reddish-yellow*; then the violet of the spectrum that appears will deviate from the red exactly as much as the disk has come closer to red; if this is just midway between yellow and red, thus *orange*, then the spectrum is pure *blue*. Orange is already more distant from white, as the full activity of the retina, than is yellow; on the other hand, its complement, blue, is just that amount nearer to white than is violet. Thus the qualitative halves of the divided activity are much less unequal to each other. They finally become quite equal when the disk becomes *red* and the spectrum is a perfect *green*. Here *red* is to be understood as Goethe's purple, that is, the true, pure red that absorbs neither yellow nor violet (very much like the color of dried-up carmine on a white china cup); not Newton's red, the prismatic, which is absolutely orange. Now this is true, pure red and is therefore just as far removed from white and black as is its complement, the perfect green. Accordingly these two colors represent the retina's activity qualitatively divided into two *equal halves*. From this can be explained their striking harmony, surpassing every other; the vigor and intensity with which they are demanded and called for; and the outstanding beauty that we assign to each of them by itself, and even more so to both together. Therefore no other colors can bear comparison with them, and I would like to call these two completely equal halves of the retina's qualitatively divided activity, red and green, χρώματα κατ' ἐξοχήν, *couleurs par excellence*,[2] because they exhibit to perfection the phenomenon of bipartition of the retina's activity. For in every other pair of colors, one of the colors is nearer to white than to black, and the other nearer to black than to white; only in this pair is this not the case. The division of the retina's activity is here preeminently *qualitative*; the quantitative, as in the other pairs, does not make itself directly felt. – Finally if our original red disk now passes into bluish-red

2. ["Colors in the superlative sense." –*Trans.*]

(violet), then the spectrum is *yellow*, and we wander through the same circle in the opposite direction.

The ratios, which follow, cannot of course be proved for the present, and we must be content to call them hypothetical.[3] Solely from perception they obtain such a decided and direct confirmation and power of conviction that hardly anyone will seriously and openly deny them. Thus Professor Anton Rosas in the first volume of his treatise on ophthalmology appropriates as his own *per fas et nefas* [4] what is mine, and straightway introduces these ratios as self-evident. (Details of this will be found in *Über den Willen in der Natur*, second edition, page 15.)[5] Just as *red* and *green* are two *completely equal* qualitative halves of the retina's activity, so *orange* is ⅔ of this activity, and its complement, *blue,* is only ⅓; *yellow* is ¾ of the full activity, and its complement, *violet,* is only ¼. From this we should not make the mistake that violet should not be ¼, because it lies midway between red, which is ½, and blue, which is ⅓. Here it is the same as in chemistry: we cannot predict from the elements the quality of the compound. Violet is the most somber of all the colors, although it originates from two colors brighter than itself, hence it also becomes brighter the moment it inclines to one side or the other. This is not the case with any other color; orange becomes brighter when it inclines to yellow and darker when it inclines to red; green becomes brighter on the yellow side and darker on the blue. Yellow, as the brightest of all colors, does the exact opposite of what is done by its complement, violet; it becomes darker whether it inclines to the orange or the green side. – From the assumption of such a relationship, expressible in whole and prime numbers, and in fact only from this can we obtain a complete explanation of why yellow, orange, red, green, blue, and violet are fixed and conspicuous points in the otherwise wholly continuous and infinitely shaded color circle, as represented by the equator of Runge's color sphere, and why they have always and everywhere been recognized by special names. Between them there are, undoubtedly, innumerable shades of color, each of which might just as well have its own name. But on what rests the prior right of these six? It is for the above-mentioned reason, namely, that, for them, the bipartition of the retina's activity is represented in the simplest

3. The statement of two experiments, which can, if necessary, serve as a proof, will be found at the end of Section 13.

4 ["By hook or by crook." –*Trans.*]

5. [*On the Will in Nature*, pp. 30–32, –*Trans.*]

fractions. It is precisely the same thing on the scale of notes, which can also be resolved into a tone that wails and howls upwards from the lower to the upper octaves through imperceptible transitions. The seven steps are marked out (and thus become a *Leiter, scala*)[6] and have received their own abstract names as prime, second, third, etc., and their own concrete names as do, ray, me, etc. The simple reason for this is that the vibrations of these very tones stand to each other in a rational numerical relation. – It is worth noting that Aristotle already surmised that there must be a numerical relation at the root of the difference between colors as well as between tones, and that, as this relation was rational or irrational, the colors turned out to be pure or not pure. He did not know, however, on what this should be based. The passage is in the book *De Sensu et Sensibili*, Chapter 3, in the middle: Ἔστι μὲν οὖν οὕτως ὑπολαβεῖν κ. τ. λ.[7] to which I observe that one has to insert τρία γάρ[8] before τὰ μέν.[9]

Note: One has not to take umbrage at the fact that, while discussing the qualitative division of the eye's activity as distinct from, and in contrast to, the merely quantitative, we nevertheless spoke of equal and unequal halves in this connection, hence of a quantitative relation. Every qualitative division is, in a subordinate sense, at the same time a quantitative. So is every chemical analysis a qualitative division of matter, in contrast to the merely quantitative mechanical division, but this qualitative division is still necessarily a quantitative one at the same time; it is a division of mass as mass, just like the mechanical.

The given explanation of color is therefore essentially as follows: *color is the qualitatively divided activity of the retina*. The difference between colors is the result of the difference between the qualitative

6. ["Gamut," "Scale." –*Trans.*]
7. [The complete passage is: "It is thus possible to believe that there are more colors than just white and black, and that their number is due to the proportion of their components; for these may be grouped in the ratio of three to two, or three to four, or in other numerical ratios (or they may be in no expressible ratio, but in an incommensurable relation of excess or defect), so that these colors are determined like musical intervals. For on this view the colors that depend on simple ratios, like the concords in music, are regarded as the most attractive, e.g., purple and red and a few others like them, few for the same reason that the concords are few, while the other colors are those that have no numerical ratios; or it may be that all are expressible in numbers, but while some are regular in ratios, others are not; and the latter, when they are not pure, have this character because they are not in a pure numerical ratio"; pp. 439b–440a, –*Trans.*]
8. ["For three." –*Trans.*]
9. ["The one." –*Trans.*]

halves into which this activity can be separated, and of their ratio to one another. These halves can be *equal* only once, and they then exhibit true red and perfect green. They can be *unequal* in innumerable ratios and hence the number of possible colors is infinite. After its appearance, every color will be followed by its *complement*, which remains behind in the eye as the physiological spectrum *for the full activity of the retina*. This happens because the nerve-like nature of the retina makes it necessary that, when the retina has been forced by the nature of the external stimulus to divide its activity into two qualitatively different halves, the half called into being by the stimulus is followed automatically by the other half after the removal of the stimulus. For the retina has the natural urge to display its activity *entirely*, and it attempts wholly to restore this after it has been split apart. The greater the portion of the retina's full activity a color is, the smaller must be its complement for this activity. In other words, the nearer an essentially and not accidently bright color is to white, the darker, the nearer to darkness, will be the spectrum appearing after it, and vice versa. As the color sphere is a continuous and uninterrupted magnitude without inner limits, and all its colors pass from one to the other by imperceptible shades, it seems that we may assume as many colors as we like, if we stop at this point of view. But it is found that, among all races and at all times, special names have been given for red, green, orange, blue, yellow, and violet, and that they have everywhere been understood to denote the same quite distinct colors, although they only rarely occur purely and perfectly in nature. They must, therefore, be known to a certain extent *a priori*, on the analogy that regular geometrical figures, which certainly do not appear perfectly in reality, yet are perfectly known and understood with all their properties. Now although these names are for the most part conferred on the actual colors only *a potiori*,[10] in other words, each color that appears is named after one of the six colors to which it comes the closest, everyone always knows how to distinguish it from the color to which that name belongs in the strictest sense, and whether and how it departs from this, for example, whether an empirically given yellow is pure or tends either to green or orange. We must therefore carry about within ourselves a standard, an ideal, an Epicurean anticipation[11] of yellow and of each color, independently of experience, with which

10. ["From preferment." –*Trans.*]

11. Anticipationem, quam appellat πρδληψιν Epicurus, i.e., anteceptam animo rei

we compare each actual color. The key to this is given to us simply and solely by the knowledge that the ratio apparently expressed by certain whole and prime numbers and into which the activity of the retina divides itself, this ratio of the two halves of the retina gives a precedence to the three previously mentioned *pairs of colors* that distinguishes them from all other colors. Accordingly, our test of the purity of a given color, e.g., whether this yellow is exactly so, or tends to green or even orange, has reference to the strict accuracy of the fraction expressed by it. The fact that we can estimate this arithmetical relation by mere sensation receives an illustration from music, the harmony of which rests on the much greater and more complicated numerical ratios of simultaneous vibrations. However, we estimate tones with extreme accuracy, and arithmetically by ear, so that every person properly qualified is in a position to state whether a note that is struck is the correct third, fifth, or octave of another. Just as the seven tones of the scale are distinguished as far as possible from countless other tones lying between them simply by the rationality of their vibration numbers, so also are the six colors, each with its own name, distinguished from innumerable others lying between them merely by the rationality and simplicity of the fraction of the retina's activity appearing in them. Just as I test the correctness of a note when tuning an instrument by striking its fifth or octave, so I test the purity of a given color by bringing about its physiological spectrum, the color of which is often easier to estimate than the given color itself. For example, I have discovered that the green of grass has a strong tendency towards yellow only from the fact that the red of its spectrum has a strong tendency towards violet. If we did not have a subjective anticipation of the six principal colors, which gives us an *a priori* standard for them, then, because their designation by their own names would be merely conventional, as is actually the case with fashionable colors, we would have no opinion on the purity of a given color and would accordingly be quite unable to understand many things. For instance, we would be unable to understand Goethe when he says of true red that it is not the ordinary scarlet which is yellowish red, but more the red of carmine, whereas this is now clear and easy to understand.

---

quandam informationem, sine qua nec intellegi quidquam nec quaeri nec disputari potest. (Cicero, *De Natura Deorum*, I, 16 [43]). ["Such an innate idea Epicurus calls 'prolepsis,' i.e., a certain form of knowledge which is inborn in the mind, and without which there can be no other knowledge, no rational thought or argument." –*Trans.*]

The follow scheme results from my discussion:

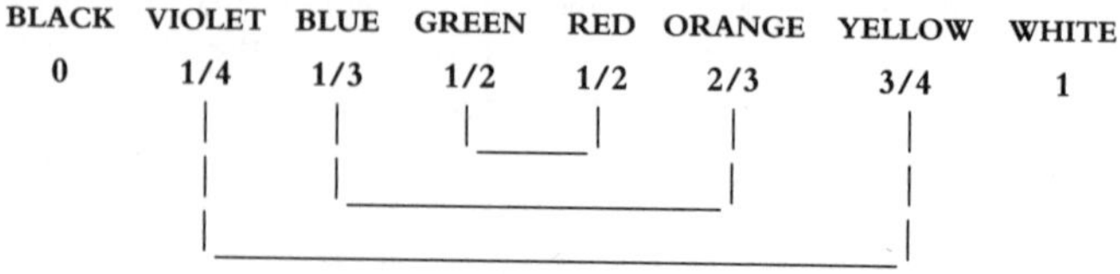

Black and white are not colors in the proper sense, as has always been recognized, because they are not fractions and so do not represent a qualitative division of the activity of the retina. They stand here merely as boundary marks for the elucidation of the subject. It is absurd, however, to assume a definite number of colors, such as seven primary colors existing outside and independent of the retina's activity and as constituting together the sum of all colors. Accordingly, true-color theory always concerns *pairs of colors*, and the purity of a given color rests on the accuracy of the fraction expressed by that color. The number of colors is infinite, yet every two opposite colors contain the elements, the full possibility of all the others. This is why, when we start from the three basic chemical colors, red, yellow, and blue, each of them has as a complement the other two in union. For color always appears as a *duality*, because it is the qualitative bipartition of the retina's activity. Therefore chromatologically, we cannot speak of individual colors, but only of *pairs of colors*, each of which contains the whole activity of the retina divided into two halves. The points of division are innumerable, and, as they are determined by external causes, they are to this extent accidental. But as soon as one half is given, the other follows necessarily as its complement. This is comparable, in music, to the keynote that is arbitrary but determines everything else. In light of what has been said, it was a double absurdity to represent the sum of all colors as consisting of an odd number. But here the Newtonians remained ever loyal to themselves, although they departed from the number fixed by their master; sometimes they assumed five, at other times three primary colors.

§6
Polarity of the Retina and Polarity Generally

With the best reasons I am now able to call the qualitatively divided activity of the retina a *polarity*, without adding a new abuse to those this concept frequently suffered during the period of Schelling's philosophy of nature. This characteristic function of the retina is thereby brought with other phenomena under *one* point of view. With these it has this in common; namely, two phenomena, *in specie* [1] opposed but *in genere* [2] identical, essentially condition each other. They do this in such a way that neither can be set up or abolished without the other, and yet they exist only in separation and contrast, and the union toward which they are constantly striving is precisely the end and disappearance of both. The polarity of the retina, however, has the characteristic that it is in time, so it is successive, and other polarity phenomena are in space and are simultaneous. Further it has the special feature that the point of indifference is displaceable, although within certain limits. The idea of a *qualitatively divided activity*, here advanced and associated with the clearest example, might even be the fundamental conception of *all polarity*, and it might be possible to bring under it magnetism, electricity, and galvanism, each of which is only the phenomenon of an activity split into two halves. These two halves condition each other, seek each other, and strive after reunion. In this sense we can then put forward an expression in Plato's words that suits them all: 'Επειδὴ οὖν ἡ φύσις δίχα ἐτμήθη, ποθοῦν ἕκαστον τὸ ἥμισυ τὸ αὑτοῦξυνήει.[3] They also come under the great Chinese contrast of *Yin* and *Yang*. The polarity of the eye, which is the most obvious to us, might even provide information about the inner essence of all polarity in many respects. By applying the notation that is customary with other polarities, we will not hesitate to assign + to red, orange, and yellow, but – to green, blue, and violet, because the brightest color and the greatest numerical fraction of the negative side, green, equals in quantity of activity only the darkest color and the smallest fraction of the positive side, red. This polar contrast must find its sharpest expression in the most perfect division into two *equal* halves. Thus red noticeably tries the eyes, and green, on the contrary, rests them. Now whether the choroidea, or even the *pigmentum nigrum*, possibly contributes in some way toward the qualitative division of the retina's activity, which might be inferred first from the obduction of the eyes of those persons who lack the ability to see colors, is something I shall return to later.

1. ["In species." –*Trans.*]
2. ["In genus." –*Trans.*]
3. ["Now when the creature was bisected, each half yearned for the half that belonged to it and united with it." *Symposium*, p. 191a, –*Trans.*]

§7
The Shaded Nature of Color

Now the following consideration appertains essentially to the color theory already advanced. It is very important for this theory, as well as for Goethe's color theory, and, taking all that has been said as well established, it is a deduction *a priori* of the essential σκιερόν [1] of color, so vigorously maintained and repeatedly urged by Goethe. As is well known, he denotes by this expression the nature of color that is akin to shade or gray, and by virtue of which the color is always brighter than black and darker than white.

In the case of the retina's qualitatively divided activity, we found the appearance of one half conditioned essentially by the *inactivity* of the other, at any rate at the same spot. But, as previously stated, *inactivity* of the retina is *darkness*. Accordingly, the appearance of the qualitative *half* of the retina's activity as color must definitely be accompanied by a certain degree of *darkness*, thus by some duskiness [*Dunkelheit*]. Now it has this in common with the *intensively* divided activity of the retina, which we previously recognized in gray or half- shade; and this very community, namely that which is there qualitative is here intensive, has been correctly understood by Goethe and denoted by the term οκιερόν. Yet there exists the following very significant difference. The fact that the activity of the retina according to *intensity* is only partial does not lead to any specific and essential variation of it, and does not involve any peculiar effect, but is merely an incidental, gradual diminution of its full activity. On the other hand, with the *qualitatively* partial activity of the retina, the activity of the one half that appears has the inactivity of the other as its essential and necessary condition, for it exists only by this contrast. From this analysis and division and its many different ratios, there arises the characteristic stimulus, the bright and cheerful impression of color, in contrast to the gray that is equal to it in clarity but somber, as is its whole specific nature, which remains always the same in spite of every variety of color. This rests simply on the fact that, in virtue of a polar separation, the vivid activity of the one half has the complete repose of the other as its support. This is the explanation of why white looks so strikingly dreary and insipid when found between colors, while gray is dismal and black is gloomy. In the same way we begin to understand why

1. "*Skieron*, (Cloudiness)," i.e., shadelike quality. –*Trans.*

the absence of the stimulus of color, hence black and white, symbolize sorrow and mourning – the former with us, the latter with the Chinese. – Because of the difference between the merely intensive and qualitative division of the retina's activity, we can very appropriately call half-shade and gray, *by way of comparison*, a merely mechanical, although infinitely fine, mixture of light with darkness. On the other hand, we can regard the color consisting in the qualitatively partial activity of the retina as a chemical combination and an intimate permeation of light and darkness. Here both neutralize one another, as it were, and by each giving up its own nature, a new product arises that has only a remote resemblance to those two, but that, on the contrary, has an outstanding character of its own. This marriage of light with darkness that necessarily emerges from the qualitative partial activity of the retina, and the phenomenon of which is color, confirms and elucidates what Goethe has perfectly, correctly, and appropriately observed, namely, that *color is essentially something shade-like*, a σκιερόν. But over and above this principle of Goethe, it also tells us that what plays the part of the σκιερόν in every color present to the eye, as the cause of its darker nature, is what afterwards appears to the eye as the ensuing spectrum; but in this spectrum itself the previously existing color now undertakes the role of the σκιερόν, because its content makes up the present deficiency.

§8
Relation of the Theory Here Advanced to Newton's Theory

In the shaded nature of colors described above, we might, to a certain extent, seek the source of Newton's confused claim "that the colors are parts of the rays of light that are dispersed by refraction."[1] He saw that color was darker than light or white; he assumed as extensive what is intensive, as mechanical what is dynamical, as quantitative what is qualitative, as objective what is subjective, by searching in light for that which was to be sought in the eye. Accordingly, he represented the ray of light as composed of seven colored rays, and, what is more, of seven rays equal in their relation to the seven intervals of the musical scale (*Spartam quam nactus es orna!*),[2] and color was supposed to

1. [*Optics*, vol. 1, 1, proposition 2, theorem 2, scholium, third edition, 1721. –*Trans.*]
2. ["Adorn hard-earned Sparta!" –*Trans.*]

be inherent in these rays as a *qualitas occulta*,[3] according to laws independent of the eye. That he selected the number seven simply and solely out of affection for the musical scale is not open to the least doubt. He had only to open his eyes to see that in the prismatic spectrum there are by no means seven colors, but only four, and that, viewed from a greater distance from the prism, the middle two, blue and yellow, overlap and thereby form green. That even now opticians enumerate seven colors in the spectrum is the height of absurdity. If we were to take this seriously, then we would be justified, forty-four years after the appearance of Goethe's color theory, to call it a barefaced lie, since by this time we have shown enough patience.

It is undeniable that, despite all this, there has been in Newton's confused theory a remote analogy, a hint of truth, and this results precisely from the point of view of our discussion. According to this point of view, instead of a divided ray of light, we have a *divided activity of the retina*, and instead of seven parts we have only two, yet again we have innumerable parts according to the way in which we consider it. For with every possible color the activity of the retina is halved, but the points of intersection, so to speak, are innumerable, and hence arise the innumerable nuances or shades of colors which are innumerable, even apart from the pale or the dark, about which we shall speak shortly. This point of view accordingly leads us from a *division of the ray of sunshine* to a *division of the retina's activity*. But this general point of view, which goes back from the observed object to the observer itself, from the objective to the subjective, can be recommended by a couple of the most brilliant examples in the history of the sciences, and can be proved to be correct. For *non aliter, si parva licet componere magnis*;[4] Copernicus replaced the movement of the whole firmament by the movement of the earth, and, in place of the absolute conditions of all things objectively recognized and set forth in ontology, the great Kant posited the cognitive forms of the subject. Γνῶθι σεαυτόν[5] appeared on the temple at Delphi!

Note: As here we have become aware of the fact that we have returned from light to the eye in our explanation of color, so that for us colors are nothing more than actions of the eye itself, appearing in polar contrasts, it may not be out of place to observe that this notion has always existed,

3. ["Occult quality." –*Trans.*]
4. ["Like this, if small things may compare with great." *Georgiea*, 4, p. 176. –*Trans.*]
5. ["Know yourself." –*Trans.*]

insofar as philosophers have always surmised that color belongs to the eye rather than to things. In particular, Locke always places color at the head of his secondary qualities of things. Generally speaking, no philosopher has ever been willing to admit that color was a real and essential constituent of bodies, while many a philosopher has preferred to admit not only extension and weight, but also every condition of a surface, such as soft and hard, smooth and rough, and, if need be, the smell and taste of a thing, as its actual constituents. On the other hand, it had to be recognized that color was something adhering to a thing and included among its properties, but at the same time that it was something found to be absolutely identical in things of the widest variety and difference, and different in things otherwise the same; hence it must be something nonessential to them. All this rendered color a difficult, perplexing, and therefore tiresome and irksome theme. For this reason an ancient author is reported by Goethe to have said: "Show a red rag to a bull and he will go mad, but the philosopher will begin to rave if one speaks about colors in a general way."[6]

An essential difference between my theory and Newton's consists in the fact that his theory (as already stated) mentions every color merely as a *qualitas occulta* (*colorifica*)[7] of one of the seven homogeneous kinds of light, gives it a name, and then leaves it at that. In this way, the specific difference of colors and the characteristic and peculiar effect of each one remain entirely unexplained. My theory, on the other hand, throws light on these characteristics and helps us to understand the reason for the specific impression and special effect of each individual color, because it tells us to recognize this as a definite portion of the retina's activity, expressed by a fraction, and further as belonging either to the + or – side of the division of this activity. Therefore it is only here that we obtain that approximation of our idea of color to its sensation, an approximation that hitherto has always been missed. For even Goethe is content with dividing colors into warm and cold, and leaves the rest to his aesthetical considerations.

The theory of color now outlined, in consequence of which color is a qualitative partial activity of the retina, leads automatically, and still more so if we consider its previously touched on analogy to Newton's mistaken theory, to the question of whether the full activity of the retina, i.e., the effect of pure light or of white, can be produced through the reunion of the two qualitative halves of the retina's

6. [*Zur Farbenlehre*, "Introduction." –*Trans.*]
7. ["Occult (color-stimulating) quality." –*Trans.*]

activity, which are revealed to us in every color and their physiological complement – just as, following Newton's assertion, the complete ray of light or white is supposed to be composed of the seven colors. To what extent this question can be answered in the affirmative in reference to both theory and practice can be better demonstrated after the theory so far advanced is supplemented by additional discussion.[8]

§9
Undivided Remainder of the Activity of the Retina

Besides the relation of the colors to one another in the color circle, complete in itself and blended by continuous transitions, we still notice, as already touched on in Section 5 above, that each color, in and of itself, has a maximum of energy that is represented by the equator on Runge's color sphere. Starting from the equator, each color is lost, on the one hand, through fading into white, and, on the other hand, through darkening into black. According to our presentation of the case, this can be explained only in the following way. While the full activity of the retina is qualitatively divided through an external stimulus, producing some color, still there can remain an unresolved part of this full activity. I am not talking about a part of the retina that can remain in undivided activity while the activity of another part is qualitatively divided. This will be discussed later. Rather, I say that the activity of the retina can *retain at the same time an undivided remainder* by being qualitatively divided for the production of color, even if this activity is spread over its entire surface. Again, this remainder can be either totally active or totally at rest, or between the two, that is to say, intensively and partially active. Accordingly, then, the color will appear pale or even darkish in many tones and shades, instead of in its full energy. In this case, we easily see that a union of the intensive with the qualitative division of the retina's activity takes place. This becomes very obvious through the fact that when we look at a color darkened and toned down by a black not essential to it, its complement appears afterwards as a spectrum toned down just as much by paleness. When we call a color vivid, energetic, or glaring, this really means, as a result of what we have said, that in its presence the entire activity of the eye is divided absolutely, without there being an undivided remainder.

8. [See Section 10 below. –*Trans.*]

§10
Production of White from Colors

I now return to the question raised above concerning the reestablishment of the retina's full activity, or of white, through the union of two opposite colors. It follows automatically that, if these colors were darkish, in other words, if a part of the retina's activity remains unresolved and at the same time also inactive, this darkness is not eliminated by that union, so gray remains. But if the colors were in full energy, in other words, if the activity of the retina was divided without remainder, or even if they were pale, that is, if their unresolved remainder was active, then as a result of our theory that considers two opposite colors as mutual complements to the retina's full activity, the division of which gave rise to them, – then, I say, the union of such colors must without doubt produce the retina's full activity and thus bring about the impression of pure light, or of white. Applied to an example, this can be expressed in the following formula:

Red=Full Activity of Retina - Green
Green=Full Activity of Retina - Red

Red+Green=Full Activity of Retina
=The Effect of Light, or of White

Even a practical demonstration of this is not difficult if we limited ourselves to colors in the strictest sense, that is, at the affectations of the eye. But then we are dealing solely with physiological colors; moreover the result of the experiment would be simply their failure to appear, and this experimental proof might seem to many people too immaterial and ethereal. For the rest, it is this: if, for example, we look at a bright red, a green spectrum will follow; if we look at green, a red spectrum follows. Now if, after looking at red, we look at once and with the same spot of the retina at a real green for just the same length of time, then both spectra fail to appear.

Only the experiment of producing white from physical, or even from chemical, colors can produce real conviction; but here there is a special difficulty. If we want to remain with these colors, then we have actually passed from the color to their cause, which, acting on the eye as stimulus, induces it to produce color, in other words, to a qualitative division of the retina's activity. Discussion of the causes of color in this sense and their relation to color in the strictest sense will occur later. Only the following is relevant here. In consequence of our theory, the production of white from two colors rests simply and solely on a physiological ground, that is to say, on the fact that there are two colors into which the retina's activity has thus separated out a physiological pair of colors. They are to be called, only and exclusively in this sense, complementary colors. Moreover, these two colors must be fully and actually reunited on the retina itself for the production of white, so that the two separated halves of the retina's activity are stimulated *simultaneously*, producing its full activity, white. But this can happen only by the two external causes, each of which excites in the eye the complementary color of the other, acting once simultaneously and yet separately on one and the same spot of the retina. Now this again is possible only under special circumstances and conditions. In the first place it cannot happen by our mixing together two chemical colors, because these then certainly act in union, but not separately. Add to this the fact that in the external material cause of color (viz., in the chemical or physical color), in the action not only for the one half of the activity of the retina but also for the repose of the other half, which appears as the σκιερόν essential to color, a concrete cause corresponding to it, a material representative, must be found. This persists as matter even after the union of opposite colors, and it continues to produce its effect, which will always give rise to gray. It, of course, gives up its role as soon as the colors have disappeared through the union of opposites, a role it played when producing them. But it now remains behind as *caput mortuum*,[1] or as their cast off mask, and as previously it contributed to the *qualitative* division of the retina's activity, it now produces an *intensively* partial activity of the retina, in other words, gray. In chemical colors, therefore, by reason of their absolutely material nature, the production of white from a pair of colors will possibly never be demonstrated, unless some special modifications supervene. I will quote an example of such production later. On the contrary, with physical colors, in fact in individual cases where we have a union of physical and chemical colors, this demonstration can be accomplished. If, however, the intermediary cloudiness in the case of physical color is of a coarse material nature, if in addition it is possibly not quite homogeneous and in places is impervious to light, like a smoked glass, a sooty smoke, a parchment, and so on, then, for the reasons mentioned, the experiment is here not a complete success. Even

1. ["Death's head." –*Trans.*]

when cloudy, however, prismatic colors provide an adequate demonstration, for here the cloudiness, as a mere hazy image, is of so delicate a nature that, if it is not actually eliminated with the union of opposite colors, either it no longer remains visible the moment it loses the significance of position by which it produced colors, or, like every aggregate cloudiness, it simply gives white. – Let us produce true red (Goethe's purple) in the objective prismatic experiment by the union of the violet of one prism with the orange of another, and let us direct green onto this from the middle of a third prism, and the spot appears *white*. Goethe himself cites this experiment (*Zur Farbenlehre*, vol. 1, p. 600, Section 556), yet he will not admit it as an example and proof of the production of white from colors, on account of his just and after all well founded polemic against Newton. But the reason that he puts forth, namely that here a threefold ray of sunlight renders invisible the gray that really exists, is in fact not convincing. For each of these three prismatic colors already contains the σκιερόν as well as the ray of sunlight. Now just as each of these three σκιερῶν is visible in each of the three colors, despite the light that is combined with it, so the whole cannot gain in brightness by three such σκιερά being united together with their three rays of light. If divisor and dividend are multiplied by the same number, the quotient is not altered. Thus it is not the increased illumination, which is balanced by the increased shade or darkness, but the contrast of the colors that here produces the impression of pure light, or of white. At the same time, and without being subject to Goethe's objection, we can more easily and distinctly carry out the following experiment. Let us turn two prismatic color spectra over each other in such a way that the violet of the first covers the yellow of the second,[2] and the blue of the first covers the orange (Newton's red) of the second; then white will also arise from the union of each one of these two pairs of colors. Moreover, since both pairs of colors lie side by side, the white spot will be twice as wide as in the former experiment. This is the thirteenth experiment of the second part of Newton's first book. Nevertheless it is certainly not in keeping with his theory; for he will now assume seven or then innumerable homogeneous rays of light (as he does alternatively, according to the occasion); but wherever we look, it is always only two colors that are covered, not seven or an infinite number. This

2. [Here Schopenhauer is using the term "spectra" in Newton's sense rather than the Goethean sense of "after-image". –*Trans.*]

experiment can be carried out even with *one* prism. Let us have two white squares on a black background, a larger and a smaller square, the latter three to four spaces under the former. Now let us look at these through the prism and move backward until the violet of the smaller square covers the yellow of the larger, and the blue of the smaller covers the orange (Newton's red) of the larger; this whole spot will then appear white. Thus with prismatic colors the production of white can be demonstrated in all three main pairs of colors. Further the experiment can be made subjectively, even with the addition of a chemical color; only then we must select a pair of colors that consists of the *most unequal* qualitative halves of the retina's activity, thus yellow and violet. Moreover, the greatest, thus essentially the brightest, half must be the chemical color and the smaller, thus the darker, must be the physical color, because only then has the persistent material σκιερόν of the chemical color insufficient mass to produce a perceptible effect. Let us look through the prism at a brilliant yellow paper, quite uniform, smooth, and spotless, on a white background. The spot where the violet fringe covers the yellow will appear completely *white*. The same thing happens when we cause the objective spectrum to fall on a yellow paper; here, however, the success is not quite so striking, because of the indistinct edges of the objective spectrum. With the other pairs of colors, this experiment is less successful; yet the brighter the chemical color, the better the results. A similar experiment, often appearing spontaneously, is provided by the lilac that adorns gardens, and frequently vases, in May. It is known also as *Syringa vulgaris*, Sirene in Lower Saxony, Nagelchen in South Germany, lila in France. The violet blue specimen produces the effect by appearing white in candle light, because its bluish violet is perfectly supplemented by the yellow tending to orange of the candlelight . Finally, white can be produced even from two chemical colors under the special provision that such colors, just like physical colors, are penetrated by light so that their σκιερόν can no longer, by itself, produce a noticeable effect as soon as it loses its significance through the disappearance of the colors by the elimination of the opposition, for example, by the union of a transparent color with a reflected color, when we cause the light to fall on a mirror of blue glass through a reddish-yellow glass. The experiment still succeeds even with *one* nontransparent color. If we throw a gold and a silver coin into a blue glass bowl, the former will appear white, and the latter blue. The same is the case with a piece of paper colored blue on both sides and reflected by polished copper; a rose illuminated merely by the light falling through a green silk curtain; and finally, also from two nontransparent chemical colors in an experiment mentioned by Helmholtz (in his thesis, *Ueber die Theorie der zusammengeseßten Farben*, 1852, p. 19). Helmholtz mentions the following way of producing white from complementary colors. A sheet of plate glass is set up vertically. A red piece of paper or wafer is put on one side, and green on the other side, in such a way that the reflected image of the green covers the red – the result is white. In all these experiments, however, the two colors must be of equal energy and equal purity. Finally, even by way of exception, all white glass appears to be white produced from the actual combination of two chemical colors found, however, in the transparent state, and I have already mentioned this in the first edition of this essay in 1816. In glassworks, as is well known, nearly all the glass turned out is originally green, and the cause of this is its iron content. Now this green, tending to a yellowish tinge, is left only in the inferior grades of glass. In order to eliminate it and produce white glass, an addition of manganese is needed, a remedy that was found empirically. By itself, however, this manganese oxide colors the glass violet red, as can be seen in the red glassy fluxes and also when, during the preparation of white glass, too much manganese is added to the green mass, and the glass assumes a reddish tinge. Examples of this include many beer glasses and, especially, English windowpanes.

The examples above may suffice to confirm what necessarily follows from my theory: that white can certainly be produced from two opposite colors. This happens only when things are so arranged that both the external, exciting causes of the two complementary colors operate *simultaneously on the same spot* of the retina, without themselves being directly blended. Now this production is a striking proof of the truth of my theory. The fact itself is never denied, but an entirely false interpretation, on the lines of Newton's erroneous theory, is attached to it, and at the same time to the fact of the physiological color spectrum. As is well known, the first is supposed to rest on the reassembly of the seven homogeneous rays of light, about which I shall speak later. For the physiological spectrum, however, the explanation that Father Scherffer gave in his *Abhandlung von den zufälligen Farben*, Vienna, 1765, and earlier in *De Coloribus accidentalibus*, 1761, shortly after Buffon's discovery of this spectrum, is still current. It starts by saying that the eye, fatigued by a long contemplation of a color, loses its susceptibility to homogeneous rays of light of this kind. The eye then experiences a sensation of white that is afterwards intuitively perceived only to the exclusion of just those homogeneous rays of color. And so the eye no longer sees this as white but experiences instead a product of the other six homogeneous rays that, together with the first color, constitute white; and hence this product is now said to be the color that appears as a physiological spectrum. But this explanation of the facts can now be seen *ex suppositis*[3] to be absurd. For after looking at violet, the eye perceives on a white (or better yet, gray) surface a *yellow* spectrum. Now this *yellow* had to be the product of the other six homogeneous lights that remained after the separation of violet, and so had to be composed of red, orange, yellow, green, blue, and indigo. Let anyone try to concoct yellow out of all of these! Above all let Mr. Pouillet try it! As a regular Newtonian true to his master, he has the effrontery to write down in his well known *Eléments de Physique* (vol. 2, p. 223) the monstrous absurdity that: "*l'orange et le vert* [thus the three chemical basic colors] *donne du jaune*."[4] One would imagine that these students of chromatics were blind, but they are only suffering from blind faith. For them, colors are really only words, mere names, or even mere numbers; they do not really know them; they do not see them. I can never forget to mention Melloni. Some twenty-five years ago, I was looking through a list of colors and their shades, compiled by him, and found a *greenish*-red mentioned![5] – From the above mixture of the six remaining colors, we shall never get anything but the color of mud instead of yellow. Moreover, yellow itself is a homogeneous ray of light; how then could it be the result of such a mixture? But the simple fact that one homogeneous ray of light is, by itself alone, the perfect complementary color of another, following it as a physiological spectrum, as yellow is of violet, blue of orange, red of green, and vice versa; even

3. ["From the assumptions." –*Trans.*]

4. ["Orange and green produce yellow." –*Trans.*]

5.* As an orthodox and imperturbable Newtonian, Humbolt speaks of color in the third volume of *Kosmos* in the following passages: pp. 86, 93, 108, 129, 169, 170, 300, and especially 496 and note 534, where he states: "The most refrangible colors in the spectrum, from *blue* to *violet*, are complementary with the less refrangible from *red* to *green* in forming white. The yellow moonlight appears white by day, because the blue atmospheric layers through which we see it furnish the complementary colors for yellow"! Page 295 indicates his qualification to give an opinion on colors, and it is here he speaks of *reddish-green*! It is just as well for him to have a monument erected during his lifetime, because after his death it will never occur to anyone to do such a thing.

this fact, I say, overthrows Scherffer's explanation. For it shows that what the eye sees on a white surface after looking continuously at a color is anything but a combination of the six remaining homogeneous light rays, but always only *one* of them, for instance yellow after looking at violet. It also cannot be assumed that, after taking away one of the seven homogeneous rays of light, the remaining six in conjunction would now produce nothing more than the color of another single light ray from their number; for we would then be assuming a cause without an effect, since the other five would not change the color of that single light ray. The inadmissible part of Scherffer's explanation even follows from the fact that the physiological color spectrum is seen not only on a white background but also perfectly well and distinctly on a completely black background, and moreover, on a shaded background; indeed even with closed eyes and covered by the hand as well. Buffon had already mentioned this, and Scherffer himself admits it in Chapter 17 of his work. Here we have a case in which, as soon as a false theory has reached a definite point, nature stands directly in its path and gives it the lie. Here too Scherffer becomes very confused and admits that this is where the greatest difficulty lies. Yet instead of being puzzled at his theory, which can never be consistent, he seizes on all kinds of wretched and absurd hypotheses, wriggles pathetically, and does not pursue the matter any further. Finally, the physiological spectrum appears on any colored surface where a conflict naturally arises between its color and the physiological color. Accordingly, when we look at a blue paper, having in our eye a yellow spectrum stimulated by a violet paper at which we have been staring, green appears, arising from the combination of the blue and the yellow. This proves irrefutably that the physiological spectrum *adds* something to the surface on which it falls, and does not *take away* something from it; for from blue we do not get green by taking away something, but by the addition of something, namely of yellow. Moreover, a white, and even more a gray or shaded, surface is obviously especially favorable to the appearance of the physiological color spectrum, because that which generally stimulates the eye's activity must also facilitate the spontaneous appearance of its qualitative halves. A gray surface that in itself excites only a part, namely an intensive part, of the eye's activity, must be particularly favorable to the already determined appearance of a qualitative part. This is also consistent with what Goethe observes (*Zur Farbenlehre*, vol. 1, p. 216), namely, that chemical color needs a white background in order to appear. – In the case of colored illumination, *shade* exhibits the complement of this color only when a second, colorless illumination enlightens it. This is due to the fact that every shade is only half shade, and this shade is therefore tinged, although only feebly, with the colored illumination. Since a colorless illumination falls on the shade, this coloring is washed and toned down to such a degree that, where it impinges on the eye, the eye is able to produce the complement of the colored illumination. – Also opposed to Scherffer's explanation of the physiological spectrum is the well known experience that we most clearly and easily see early in the morning, immediately after waking up. Precisely at this time the retina is at its maximum strength as a result of a long rest. It is, therefore, least likely to become fatigued by continuously looking at a color for several seconds, and to become dead and indifferent to the point of complete insensitivity to this color. – All that I have said here shows irrefutably that the physiological spectrum is created out of the retina's own power; it belongs to the retina's action; it is not an impression of a white surface that proves to be defective and abortive through the retina's exhaustion. I have had to make a thorough refutation of Scherffer's explanation, because it is still accepted as valid by Newtonians. I mention with regret that even Cuvier has advanced it in his *Anatomie comparée* (lecon 12, article 1), whereupon he announces it as his own new invention, and for which he has been commended in Jameson's *Edinburgh New Philosophical Journal*, April–September, 1828, page 190. The fact that ordinary compendium writers are forever harping on this explanation is hardly worth mentioning; and the fact that, even in the year 1853, Professor Dove favors us with it in his *Darstellung der Farbenlehre* (p. 157) need not surprise us in a book of that sort.

The entire doctrine of *complementary colors* held by all present day physicists and all their gossip about it rest on Scherffer's theory. As they are truly incurable, they always understand the matter *objectively* in the Newtonian sense. Accordingly, their frequently mentioned *complement* refers always only to the Newtonian spectrum of seven colors and indicates a part of these, separated from the rest, which are thereby supplemented to compose white light as the sum of all the homogeneous rays of light, as is expounded at some length by Pouillet in his *Eléments de Physique* (vol. 2, Section 393). But this interpretation of the matter is fundamentally false and absurd, and it is unpardonable that, forty-four years after Goethe's color theory and forty years after my theory, it still enjoys a great reputation and is imposed on young people.

On the other hand, it is undeniable that Goethe went too far and strayed from the path of truth by unconditionally denying the production of white from colors. However, he did this simply because he constantly had in mind Newton's erroneous teaching, and quite rightly contended that the aggregation of colors does not lead to light, for each color is related to darkness as well as to light. Thus, by such denial, he was particularly anxious to maintain the σκιερόν of color, although he knew that the colors physiologically required were destroyed when blended. He explained this primarily from the mixture of the three basic colors in a chemical sense, and he wished to maintain that gray was the real and unconditional result. Because he had not gone right to the ultimate ground of all color phenomena, which is purely physiological, but had achieved his goal through the highest law of all *physical* colors, their true and ultimate ground remained hidden from him. This ground is to the effect that opposite colors, when combined, are eliminated, because they are the qualitative halves of the retina's activity, which is thus again combined. In the same way, the real ground and inner essence of that σκιερόν inseparable from color, and so emphatically stressed by him, also remained hidden from him. This is nothing but the appearance of the repose of the inactive half of the retina's activity, and consequently it must completely disappear through the reunion of the two halves. Finally gray, which chemical colors leave behind with their disappearance through the union of opposites, is not related to the colors themselves but only to the material condition in this, their crudely material cause, and can be called contingent with reference to the colors as such. If one wanted to reproach Goethe for this misunderstanding, which is found in an extensive work that uncovers so many errors and teaches so many truths, it would be, moreover, the greatest injustice and ingratitude. The true reason for the production of white from two colors could be revealed only as the result of my theory. *Multi pertransibunt et augebitur scientia.*[6]

On the other hand, however, we cannot possibly maintain that Newton has hit upon the truth on this point. For although it has to be admitted that he teaches in a general way that white can be produced from colors, yet the sense in which he says so, namely the doctrine

6. ["Many will examine it thoroughly, and knowledge will be increased." –*Trans.*]

that the seven colors are the basic constituents of light, which is recomposed through their combination, is fundamentally false. The physiological contrast of colors, upon which rests their whole nature, and with regard to which alone the production of white, or of the effect of light, results from colors, in fact from *two* colors or any arbitrary *pair of colors*, and not from seven definite colors – such a contrast, I say, was forever unknown to him. In fact he was totally unaware of it, and so was unaware also of the true nature of color. Moreover, the production of white from two colors demonstrates the impossibility of its production from seven. Therefore we cannot say in Newton's favor more than that he accidentally pronounced a judgment that came near the truth. But because he expressed this in a false sense and for the purpose of a false theory, the experiments by which he tried to illustrate it are, for the most part, insufficient and false. It was precisely in this way that he led Goethe to deny too much in contradicting this false theory. And so we have the curious case where the true and real fact of the production of the impression of light or of white through the combination of colors (we must here leave it indefinite whether two or seven) is affirmed by Newton from an incorrect ground and for the purpose of a false theory but is denied by Goethe in connection with an otherwise correct system of the facts. If this were true in the Newtonian sense, or if Newton's theory in general were correct, then, in the first place, every combination of two basic colors assumed by it would inevitably give us at once a color brighter than each of them alone, because the combination of two homogeneous parts of white light that is divided into these would already be a step back toward the restoration of this white light. But this is not for one moment the case. Thus, if we bring together in pairs the three fundamental colors in the chemical sense and of which all the rest are composed, then blue with red gives violet that is darker than either of these two; blue with yellow gives green that is indeed much darker than the latter, although it is somewhat brighter than the former; yellow with red gives orange that is brighter than the latter but darker than the former. Already we see here a really adequate refutation of Newton's theory.

But its correct, factual, conclusive, and inescapable refutation is the achromatic refractor; and precisely on this account Newton very consistently regards such a thing as impossible. If white light consists of seven different kinds of light, each of which has a different color and at the same time a different refrangibility, then the degree of refraction and the color of the light are of necessity inseparably associated. Thus where light is *refracted*, it must then appear as *colored*; however much the refraction may be distorted, varied, and complicated; only so long as all the rays are not again brought together into a heap and thus, according to Newton's theory, white is recomposed, an effect of refraction then at the same time being ended, and so everything again is back in its place. Now when the invention of achromatism revealed the very opposite of this result, the Newtonians in their embarrassment seized on an explanation that, with Goethe, we feel tempted to regard as senseless rubbish; for with the best will in the world, it is very difficult to attribute to it any intelligible meaning, that is to say, something that can to a certain extent be represented in intuitive perception. So besides the color refraction, there is supposed to occur a *color dispersion* different from it; and by this is to be understood the distance of the separated colored lights from one another, their dispersion, which is the most immediate *cause* of the lengthening of the spectrum. But this is, *ex hypothesi*,[7] the *effect* of the different refrangibility of those colored rays. Now if this so-called dispersion, namely, the lengthening of the spectrum and thus of the sun's image after refraction, rests on the fact that light consists of different colored lights, each of which has, by its nature, a different refrangibility, that is to say, is refracted in a different angle, then this definite refrangibility of each ray of light must always and on all occasions adhere to it as an essential and inseparable property. Hence the individual homogeneous ray of light must always be refracted in the same way, just as it is always colored in the same way. For Newton's homogeneous light ray and its color are absolutely one and the same; it is simply a colored ray and nothing else. Consequently, where there is a ray, there is also its color; and where there is color, there too is its ray. If *ex hypothesi* it lies in the nature of every such differently colored ray to be refracted at a different angle, then its color will also accompany it in this and every angle; consequently with each refraction the different colors must appear. And so in order to attribute any sense to the Newtonians' favorite explanation that "two different kinds of refracting media can refract light with equal intensity but disperse colors in varying degree," we must assume that, while crown-glass and flint-glass

7. ["According to the hypothesis." –*Trans.*]

refract light as a whole, hence white light with equal intensity, yet the parts that make up this whole light are refracted by flint-glass differently from the way in which they are by crown-glass and thus alter their refrangibility. A hard nut to crack! – Moreover, they must alter their refrangibility in such a way that, with the use of flint- glass, the most refrangible rays receive a still more intense refrangibility, whereas the least refrangible rays obtain an even smaller refrangibility. Thus the flint-glass increases the refrangibility of certain rays and at the same time diminishes the refrangibility of certain others and that; nevertheless, the whole light, which consists of these rays alone, retains its previous refrangibility. Despite all this, this very difficult dogma is held in universal credit and respect; and from the optical writings of all nations we can see, even at the present day, how seriously the difference between refraction and dispersion is discussed. Now let us turn to truth!

The nearest and most essential cause of achromatism that is produced by means of the combination of a convex lens from crown- glass and a concave lens from flint-glass must be a *physiological* cause, like every production of white from colors. It must be the production of the retina's *full* activity at those places that are affected by physical colors, since here two colors, certainly not seven, namely two colors that together make up that activity, are brought onto each other; and so a pair of colors is again united. In the present case this is brought about objectively or physically in the following manner. Through a refraction occurring twice in opposite directions (by means of concave and convex glasses), there results the opposite color phenomenon, on the one hand, a yellowish-red band with a yellow edge and, on the other hand, a blue band with a violet edge. This refraction, occurring twice in opposite directions, at the same time brings these two colored bands over each other in such a way that the blue band covers the yellowish-red and the violet edge covers the yellow. In this way these two physiological pairs of colors, namely one of $1/3$ and $2/3$ and the other of $1/4$ and $3/4$ of the retina's full activity, are again united; consequently, colorlessness or achromatism is again produced. This, then, is the *nearest* cause of achromatism.

Now what is the *more remote* cause? Thus as the required dioptric result, namely a surplus of refraction that remains *colorless*, is produced through the flint-glass, acting in the opposite direction, and is able to neutralize with a considerably smaller refraction the color phenomenon of the crown-glass through an opposite color phenomenon that is just as wide, because its own color bands and edges are originally considerably wider than those of the crown-glass, the question then arises of how it is that two different kinds of refracting media with equal refraction give such a very different width of color phenomenon. A very satisfactory account of this can be given in accordance with Goethe's theory, if we follow it up in more detail and more clearly than did he himself. His derivation of the prismatic color phenomenon from his highest principle, which he calls the primary phenomenon, is perfectly correct; only he has not reduced it to sufficiently specific details, whereas without a certain amount of acribology in such things no satisfaction is felt. He quite rightly explains this color-band phenomenon accompanying refraction from a subsidiary image that accompanies the main image displaced by refraction. But he has not specifically determined the position and mode of action of this subsidiary image and does not make this clear by a sketch. Indeed, he speaks throughout of only *one* subsidiary image, and the result is that we have to assume that not merely the light or illuminating image, but also the darkness surrounding it, undergoes a refraction. I must, therefore, supplement what he has said, in order to show how the varying width of the colored-band phenomenon really arises with equal refraction but with different refracting substances. The Newtonians denote this width by the meaningless expression of a difference of refraction and dispersion.

Let us first say a word on the origin of these subsidiary images that accompany the main image in refraction. *Natura non facit saltus*;[8] so runs the law of the continuity of all changes by virtue of which no transition in nature occurs with complete abruptness in space, or time, or in the degree of any property. Now when light enters and emerges from a prism, it is twice diverted suddenly from its straight path. Now are we to suppose that this happens so abruptly and with such sharpness that the light does not suffer the slightest admixture with the surrounding darkness, but that, turning through considerable angles in this darkness, it yet preserves its edges in the sharpest possible manner – so that it comes through in wholly unalloyed purity and remains completely whole? Is it not more natural to assume that, in the first as well as in the second refraction, a very small part of this mass of light does not take up the new alignment rapidly enough and so becomes somewhat detached, and now, as it were, remembering as an afterthought the path just forsaken, it accompanies the main image

8. ["Nature makes no leaps." –*Trans.*]

as a subsidiary one that hovers somewhat above it after one refraction, and somewhat under it after the other? For this reason it has also been observed that, with every refraction of light, there is necessarily associated a toning down or diminution of light (Birnbaum, *Reich der Wolken*, p. 61). Here one might think of the polarization of light by means of a mirror that reflects one part of the light and lets through the other part. But the essential thing is that light refracted in its surrounding darkness enters into so intimate a blending that this no longer calls into existence the merely intensive division of the retina's activity, as half shades do for example, but also the qualitative division of this activity.

The adjoining figure shows more particularly how, from the effect of those two subsidiary images that fall off with prismatic refraction, there arise, in accordance with Goethe's fundamental law, the four prismatic colors that alone really exist, and not seven.

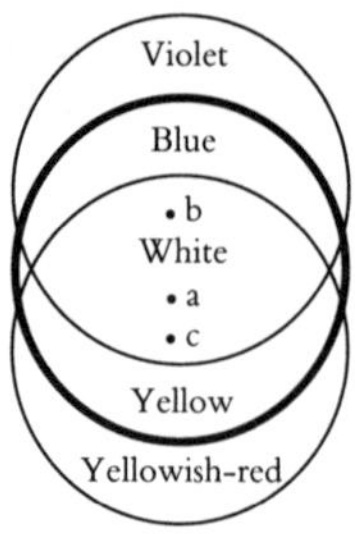

This figure represents a white paper disk, some four inches in diameter, stuck on black unglazed paper, as seen through the prism from a distance of about three paces, and as depicted in nature and not in accordance with Newtonian fictions. Now in order to know what we are talking about, you must convince yourself by personal observation. By holding the prism before your eyes and by stepping now nearer, now further away, you will then perceive the two subsidiary images almost at once, and you will see how they follow your movement and deviate more or less from the main image, and how they shift over each other. If you step back very much farther, then blue and yellow spread over one another, and you enjoy the extremely edifying spectacle of seeing Newton's *homogeneous* green, the pure original green, composed from them. – Generally speaking, prismatic experiments can be carried out in two different ways; either so that refraction precedes reflection, or vice versa. The former is the case when the sun's image passes through the prism and falls on the wall; the latter is the case when we observe a white image through the prism. This latter method is not only less troublesome to carry out, but also shows the actual phenomenon more clearly. This is partly due to the fact that the effect of refraction directly reaches the eye, and we thus have the advantage of receiving the effect at firsthand, whereas with the other method we receive it secondhand, namely after reflection from the wall has taken place. It is also due partly to the fact that the light here proceeds directly from a near object that is sharply defined and not dazzling, whereas with the first method it is the image of a body twenty million miles away, correspondingly large and radiating its own light, that passes directly through the prism. Thus the white disk here depicted (whose place is taken by the sun in the first method) shows quite clearly the two subsidiary images that accompany it and that have arisen as the result of a double refraction displacing it upwards. The subsidiary image arising from the first refraction, which takes place when the light enters the prism, trails behind and thus remains with its extreme edge still in darkness and covered over by it. The other subsidiary image, on the contrary, which results from the second refraction, hence when the light emerges from the prism, moves forward rapidly and for this reason is drawn over the darkness. The effect of both, however, extends, although more feebly, to *that* portion of the main image that is toned down by their loss; hence only *that* portion of it that remains covered by the *two* subsidiary images, and thus retains its full light, appears white. On the other hand, where *one* subsidiary image *alone* is in conflict with the darkness, or the main image that is somewhat weakened by the loss of this image and is already impaired by the darkness, colors result, and moreover in accordance with Goethe's law. Therefore, we see violet arise on the upper part where *one* subsidiary image alone advances and is rapidly drawn over the black surface; but under it we see blue where the main image, although weakened by loss, is operating. On the lower portion of the image, however, we see the single subsidiary where the individual secondary image remains in darkness and yellowish-red appears; but over this we see yellow where the weakened main image already shines through. In just the same way, the rising sun appears yellowish-red at first, when covered by the lower and denser atmospheric layers, but appears yellow when it has reached the more rarefied atmosphere. Just because, according to this interpretation, it is not the white disk alone that produces colors, since darkness operates as a second factor, the phenomenon of color turns out much better when the white disk is fixed on a black background than when it is fixed on a light gray background.

After this explanation of the prismatic phenomenon, it will not be difficult for us to understand, at any rate in a general way, why, with equal refraction of light, some refracting media, like flint-glass, give a wider colored band, while others, like crown- glass, give a narrower band; or in the language of the Newtonians, what gives rise to the lack of uniformity in light refraction and color dispersion. *Refraction* is the distance of the main image from its line of incidence; *dispersion*, on the other hand, is the distance of the two subsidiary images from the main image that occurs here. But now we find this *accidental property* existing in varying degrees in different kinds of light- refracting substances. Accordingly, two transparent bodies can have equal power of refraction; in other words, they can deflect the image of light passing through them an equal amount from its line of incidence. Nevertheless, the *subsidiary images* that cause the phenomenon of color can deviate from the *main image* more with refraction through one body than with refraction through another.

Now in order to compare this account of the facts with the Newtonian explanation of the phenomenon, which has been so often repeated and is analyzed above, I select the expression of the latter, which is given in the following words in the *Münchner Gelehrten Anzeigen* of 27 October 1836 after the "Philosophical Transactions": "Different transparent substances refract the various homogeneous rays of light in very unequal proportion;[9] so that the spectrum produced by different refracting media, and moreover in similar circumstances, acquires a very different extension." – If the lengthening of the spectrum generally results from the unequal refrangibility of the homogeneous rays of light, then it must everywhere turn out according to the degree of refraction, and therefore greater lengthening of the image could result only from the greater power of refraction of a particular medium. Now if this is not the case, but two media have equal refractive power, one giving a longer and the other a shorter spectrum, this proves that the lengthening of the spectrum is not the direct effect of *refraction*, but merely the effect of an *accident* accompanying refraction. Now the subsidiary images here arising are such an

9. Yet the sum of these, namely white light, in equal proportion! I add this as a supplement.

accident; these may very well deviate more or less from the main image with equal refraction, according to the nature of the refracting substance.

§11
The Three Kinds of Division of the Activity of the Retina in Combination

For the sake of completeness, I must still observe that as the deviation of color from its highest energy, towards either paleness or darkness, is a union of the *qualitative* with the *intensive* division of the activity of the retina, in the same way the *extensive* division is associated with the qualitative, because with an external stimulus, one part of the retina produces one color and another part another color. We know that after the cessation of the stimulus the two required colors appear on each spot as spectra. With the ordinary use of the eye, all three kinds of division of the retina's activity often are achieved simultaneously and in combination.

If one wishes to raise a difficulty by saying that, according to my theory, when looking at a multicolored surface, the activity of the retina is distributed simultaneously in a hundred places in very different proportions, then let that person reflect that, when listening to the harmony of a large orchestra, or to the rapid runs of a virtuoso, the eardrum and auditory nerve are moved now in simultaneous vibrations and then in vibrations that most rapidly succeed one another, according to different numerical ratios. The intellect arithmetically grasps and assesses all these ratios; it receives the aesthetic effect from them and notices every deviation from the mathematical accuracy of a tone. One will then find that I have not attributed too much to the far more perfect sense of sight.

A particular and, to some extent, abnormal phenomenon is worth mentioning here. It is certainly incompatible with Scherffer's interpretation and so contributes to its refutation; but even by mine it requires a special explanation. If on a large colored surface there are some smaller colorless spots, then when the physiological spectrum produced by the colored surface subsequently appears, these smaller spots will no longer remain colorless but will appear in the previously existing color of the whole surface itself, although they have not been in any way affected by its complement. For example, after looking at a green wall with small gray windows, there follows as a spectrum a red wall, not with gray, but with green windows. According to my theory, we have to explain this from the fact that while after a definite qualitative half of its activity had been produced on the whole retina by the colored surface, a few small spots, however, remained excluded from this stimulation. When this external stimulus ceases, the complement of that half of activity, excited by the stimulus, now appears as a spectrum. The spots that remained excluded from this stimulus then enter, in a consensual way, into that qualitative half of activity existing previously since they now imitate, as it were, what was previously done by the whole of the rest of the retina even though they alone, through the non-appearance of the stimulus, were excluded from it; consequently they go through the exercise afterwards, so to speak.

§12
Concerning Some Injuries and an Abnormal Condition of the Eye

Here we might also mention that those spectra produced by mechanical shock to the eye and those produced by glare and dazzle are to be regarded as of the same kind, differing only in degree. They can be appropriately called pathological spectra, for just as the former result from obvious injury, so the latter are phenomena of a transitory disorganization of the retina's activity, produced by overstimulation. This activity, thrown off its balance as it were, is then divided convulsively in one way or another and exhibits the phenomena described by Goethe (*Zur Farbenlehre*, vol. 1, p. 15). When looking at brightness a dazzled eye has a red spectrum, and when looking into darkness, a green spectrum. This is because its activity is divided by the force of the powerful stimulation, and now one or the other half appears, according to the external circumstance.

Injury to the eye, as opposed to glare, is the strain of the eye in faint light. With glare the stimulus from outside is too powerful; with strain in faint light the stimulus is too weak. Through the deficient external stimulus of light, the activity of the retina is intensively divided, and only a small part of it is actually excited. Now this is increased by voluntary strain, for example by reading, so an intensive part of the activity is excited without stimulus, entirely by inner strain. In order to make plain the harmfulness of this, I cannot think of any simile but an obscene one. That is to say, it harms in the same way as onanism and generally any excitation of the genitals that arises through mere fantasy and without the influence of a naturally appropriate external stimulus, and that is more ravishing than the actual natural satisfaction of the sexual drive.

Only through my theory do we really first understand why artificial illumination from candlelight fatigues the eye more than daylight. The light of a flame gives everything a reddish- yellow illumination (hence also blue shadows). It follows that as long as we see by candlelight, only two-thirds of the retina's activity is stimulated and endures the entire strain of vision, while approximately one-third remains idle. This must strain the eye in a way similar to the use of ground-glass before one eye. In fact it does so even more, because the division of the retina's activity is not simply intensive, but is also qualitative, and the retina remains without repose for a long time. The same is true of its impulse to produce the complement, an impulse that it satisfies at each occasion by immediately coloring every faintly illuminated shadow. It was accordingly a good suggestion for making night illumination similar to daylight by using blue glasses lightly tinted by violet. From my own experience I recommend glasses not too dark or too thick; otherwise the result is only the semblance of faint light. Moreover, one should see Parrot, *Traité de la manière de changer la lumière artificielle en une lumière semblable à celle du jour*, (Strasburg, 1791).

An additional proof of the subjective nature of color, namely that it is a function of the eye itself, consequently related immediately first to this and secondarily and mediately to objects, is given to us, to begin with, by the *daguerreotype*, which in its purely objective way reproduces everything visible of bodies, but not color. An even more striking proof is furnished by those cases of people that are admittedly rare, yet occur from time to time. These people do not perceive color, and their retinas accordingly lack the capacity for the qualitative division of their activity. Thus they see only the gradations of light and dark, and consequently the world appears to them like a black and white picture, or a copper engraving, or a daguerreotype. Their retinas are deprived of that characteristic stimulus that provides color for us. An example of this is found in the sixty-seventh volume of the *Philosophical Transactions of* 1777, where (on page 260) a detailed account is given of three brothers named Harris, all of whom saw no colors. In the following volume there is an essay by Janus Scott, who saw no colors, a defect that several members of his family also shared. Suffering from the same defect was Doctor Unzer, who was famous in his day and lived in Hamburg. He was most concerned to hide his color blindness as far as possible, because due to it he had an obvious difficulty with diagnosis and semiotics. In order to get to the bottom of the matter, his wife once covered her face with blue cosmetics, and his only comment was that she had applied too much rouge. I am indebted to a painter named Demiani for this account. Forty years ago he was the inspector of the Dresden gallery, and the situation had come to his knowledge because he painted a portrait of Unzer's wife. Unzer confessed to him the reason why he was unable to offer any criticism on colors and coloring. Herr von Zimmermann affords yet another example of this kind; he was living in Riga at the beginning of the [nineteenth] century. The publisher of this work[1] vouches for the following account, because he knew the man himself, and also quotes Albanus, the head of the upper school, who was his master. Colors did not exist for this Herr von Zimmermann; he saw everything in black, white, and all the shades and nuances of gray. He played billiards very well, and since in Riga this game is played with yellow and red balls, he was well able to distinguish them, because the red ball appeared to him to be much darker. (According to my theory, with pure colors, red for him must have been half as dark again as yellow.) Someone carried out an experiment with him that, in regard to my theory, could not have been more fortunately devised. He wore a red uniform; a green uniform was laid out for him instead. He noticed absolutely nothing, put the green uniform on, and was on the point of going out on parade in it. Naturally, pure red and pure green must have been for him as identical as half and half. His retina therefore completely lacked the capacity for dividing its activity qualitatively. – Much less rare are those people who only see colors very imperfectly because they recognize but a few of them, and not the majority. In my own experience I have come across three such cases. They were least able to distinguish red and green, for the reason just given. That such an achromatic defect can appear temporarily is seen from an essay by Thomas Clemens, "*Farbenblindheit während der Schwangerschaft, nebst einigen Erörterungen über Farbenblindheit im allgemeinen*," to be found in the *Archiv für physiologische Heilkunde vom Jahre 1858*. (Compare also George Wilson, *Researches on Colour Blindness*, Edinburgh, 1855.)

1. J. F. Hartknoch in the year 1815.

§ 13
On the External Stimuli that Stimulate the Qualitative Division of the Activity of the Retina

Hitherto we have considered colors in the strictest sense, that is to say, as conditions and affections of the eye. This consideration is the first and essential part of the theory of colors in the strictest sense, which, as such, must be the basis of all further investigations of colors, and with which these investigations must always remain in agreement. To this first part is to be added the second; namely, a consideration of the causes that, as stimuli acting on the eye from without, do not produce the undivided activity of the retina in stronger or weaker degrees, as do pure light and white, but that always produce only a qualitative half of this activity. Goethe has quite correctly and appropriately separated these external causes into two classes, namely into chemical and physical colors, that is to say, into those permanent colors inherent in bodies and those merely temporary colors arising through some special combination of light with transparent media. Now if their distinction is to be indicated by one perfectly general expression, then I would say that physical colors are those causes of stimulation of a qualitative half of the retina's activity that are comprehensible to us as such. So we see that, although we are not in agreement concerning their mode of operation, this mode must yet be subject to certain laws that exist under the most varied circumstances and in the case of the most varied materials, so that the phenomenon can always be referred to it. Chemical colors, on the other hand, are those for which this is not the case but recognize their causes without in any way comprehending the manner of their special action on the eye. For although we know that this or that chemical precipitate, for example, gives this definite color and is to this extent its cause, we still do not know the cause of the color *as such*; we do not know the law as a result of which it appears here; rather, its appearance is known only *a posteriori*, and to this extent it is for us accidental. On the other hand, we know the cause of physical colors *as such*; we know the law of their appearance. Therefore our knowledge of them is not tied to certain materials but holds good of any material; so, for example, yellow occurs as soon as light is refracted through a cloudy or opaque medium, and this may be a parchment, a liquid, a smoke, or the prismatic subsidiary image. – Even black and white exist physically as well as chemically; physical black is darkness, and physical white is perfectly cloudy opaqueness. In consequence of what I have said, we can call *physical* colors *comprehensible*, but *chemical* colors *incomprehensible*. By reducing chemical colors to physical in some sense, the second part of the theory of colors would be completed. Newton has done the very opposite of this and reduced physical colors to chemical by teaching that in refraction the white ray is split up into seven unequally refrangible parts and that these had a violet, indigo, etc., color just by accident.

I will say something more about chemical color later. Here I will deal with physical color in the first instance. As the external stimulus of the retina's activity is ultimately always light, it must be possible to demonstrate, for the modification of this activity, in which the sensation of color consists, a modification of light exactly corresponding to it. This is the *punctum controversiae*[1] between Newton and Goethe, which is to be settled in the last resort by a display of facts and experiments and a correct judgment of them. Now if we take into consideration what was explained above in Chapter 2 about the necessary parallelism between cause and effect, then we will have no doubt that the more precise knowledge of the effect to be explained, hence of color as physiological fact – knowledge gained by what has been said so far – puts us in a position to settle something about its external causes, for which we have been searching independently of any experimental investigation, and hence to this extent *a priori*. This is principally as follows:

(1) The colors themselves, their mutual relations, and the laws by which they appear all reside within the eye itself, and they are all only a special modification of the retina's activity. The external cause can act only as stimulus, as the occasion for exciting this activity; hence it can act only in a very subordinate way. With the production of color in the eye, in other words, with the stimulation of the polarity of the retina, the external cause can play only the same part as friction can play in the production of electricity lying dormant in a body, that is to say, in the separation of +E and –E. Colors cannot in any way exist in a definite number somewhere outside the eye in a purely objective way; outside of the eye they cannot have definite laws and mutual relations and be offered to the eye ready-made. If, in spite of all this, there is a desire to establish an agreement between my theory and Newton's, then such an unhappy idea could only be made on the-

1. ["Point of controversy." –*Trans.*]

most marvelous *harmonia praestabilita*[2] ever resorted to by a human head in its speculative embarrassment. In consequence of such a *harmonia*, certain colors, although originating in the eye according to the laws of its functions, just like all the other innumerable colors, must already be in light itself, and indeed in its constituents, have causes expressly prepared and, as it were, arranged for this.

(2) Every color is the qualitative half of the retina's full activity, to which it is supplementary through another color, its complement. Consequently there are only pairs of colors and no individual colors; hence we cannot assume seven colors, an odd number, actually existing separately.

(3) Colors form a continuous circle inside of which there are no boundaries, no fixed points, like the equator of Runge's color sphere, described previously in Chapter 5. Each color results from the division of this circle into two halves, and its complementary opposite is given at once. The two together always contain *potentialiter* the whole circle.[3] Thus colors are infinite in number; so we certainly cannot assume either seven or any other definite number of fixed colors. Three pairs of colors are specially distinguished simply by the rational proportion, easily understood and expressed in simple numbers, in which the retina's activity is divided. For this reason, these pairs are everywhere and always expressed by names of their own, but, except for this, there is no other reason, because, after all, they have no advantage over the others.

(4) To the infinite number of possible colors arising from the divisibility of the retina's activity and modifiable in endless ways there must also correspond in the external cause, acting as stimulus, a modifiability just as infinite and capable of the most delicate and imperceptible changes. But this in no way establishes the assumption of seven or any other definite number of homogeneous rays of light as parts of white light, each of which stands out by itself fixed and rigid, but which, united with one another, could never produce anything but a return to colorlessness. When the thread and sequence of his argument demand it, I am well aware that Newton sometimes asserts that the seven homogeneous rays of light are, at bottom, meant only in jest; that they are by no means homogeneous but extremely complex and composed of an infinite number of rays that are really and

2. ["Preestablished harmony." –*Trans.*]
3. ["Potentiality." –*Trans.*]

truly homogeneous. Now, even expressed here, this might at most save the homogeneous rays of light from the requirement of this paragraph, but the same argument destroys them all the more certainly in the next. For, not to mention that they now exist only like Democritus' atoms, it follows that each homogeneous ray of light, that is to say, each actual primary color, is related to white as an *infinitely small* fraction is to one. In this way it completely vanishes into darkness and becomes invisible. – On the other hand, Goethe's theory satisfies most perfectly the requirement stated here. For something dull and cloudy that can be now on one side of light, now on the other; that can thus be in innumerable degrees at one moment more opaque, at another more transparent; and, finally, that can be illuminated from both sides unequally in the most varied proportions, again gives us in the cause the same infinite modifiability that we had found in the effect.

(5) We have found that the σκιερόν [4] essential to color, or its shaded nature, is set up in the eye, and that one-half of the retina's activity presupposes the repose of the other half, the expression of which is precisely this σκιερόν. We have compared its intimate association with light, which through this necessity appears in color, to a chemical mixture of light and darkness. This σκιερόν must be found again outside the eye, represented [*repäsentirt*] in some way in the external cause. Now on this point, Newton's theory that color is always one-seventh of the whole of light would be extremely unsatisfactory, since it recognizes color as something of less brightness than white, yet to an exaggerated extent in that all colors (with minor differences) are each related to white in brightness as one to seven, or, at any rate, one to six. But we know that even the weakest and darkest of all colors, namely violet, is related to white as one to four; blue as one to three; green and red as one to two; and yellow at least as three to four. In the previous paragraph it has already been explained how sad is the plight of Newton's theory, if an infinite number of homogeneous rays of light is assumed, as this truly esoteric theory teaches, instead of seven. – On the other hand, the primary phenomenon advanced by Goethe answers the requirement regarding the σκιερόν most perfectly and satisfactorily. Goethe represents color as resulting from the most intimate combination of light and darkness. An obscured light stimulates yellow in the eye; and illuminated darkness stimulates blue. Neither, however, can happen directly – because in

4. ["Cloudiness," i.e., shade-like quality. –*Trans.*]

this case dimness, faint light, gray, or intensive division of the retina's activity would result – but by means of the intervention of a third thing, of something dull and cloudy that becomes, as it were, the *menstruum* [5] of the chemical penetration of light and darkness, and this now produces the polarity of the eye, in other words, the qualitative division of its activity. After Goethe had appropriately described the *physiological* contrast of colors in all its phenomena, he put forward yellow and blue as a *physical* contrast arising from opposite causes: yellow, through something dull and cloudy checking the light to the eye; blue, by the eye looking into darkness through an illuminated cloudy object. Now this physical contrast is quite correct as long as we understand it as the universal expression for two principal relations of all physical colors, and here regard blue and yellow as representatives of two classes, so to speak, of cold and warm colors. But if we wish to interpret it in the strictest sense and assume a physical contrast actually existing between yellow and blue, then we inevitably are surprised at the incongruity between the contrast of physiological colors with the contrast of physical, since the proper contrast of blue is orange and of yellow is violet; and it had to be assumed that the relation, existing between colors in the strictest sense, would again have to be found between their causes lying outside the eye, in accordance with the Aristotelian principle quoted above: τῶν ἐναντίων τὰ ἐναντία αἴτια (*contrariorum contrariae sunt causae*)[6]: *De Generatione et Corruptione*, Book II, Chapter 10. It certainly is so, and this incongruity is merely apparent. For more closely considered, the same degree of cloudiness that stimulates pure blue when drawn and illuminated before darkness gives not yellow but orange when, conversely, it impedes the light. In just the same way, one and the same degree of cloudiness will always give two opposite and mutually complementary colors under opposite circumstances as regarding light and darkness. That this must be so is the *a priori* result of the following consideration. The color required and subsequently following as spectrum is the complement of the given color; therefore it must fall short of the eye's full activity as much as the given color has fallen short; in other words, it must contain precisely as much darkness, σκιερόν, as the other contains light. Now in the case of all physical colors on the pos-

5. ["Solvent." –*Trans.*]

6. "Contrary effects demand contraries as their causes." [Aristotle, *De Generatione Corruptione*, 2, ch. 10, p. 460a. –*Trans.*]

itive side (i.e., all those lying between yellow and red), cloudiness is the cause of their darkness, because it impedes the light. Conversely, in the case of all colors on the negative side, cloudiness is the cause of their brightness, since it reflects the incident light that would otherwise be lost in the darkness. Therefore, the same cloudiness, in opposite circumstances, must cause precisely as much brightening in one case as it causes darkening in the reverse case. As it is shown that each color must contain as much brightness as its complement contains darkness, so, with opposite illumination, the same cloudiness will necessarily give the two colors that are required and supplementary. Here, I ask the reader to note carefully we have a perfect demonstration, *a priori,* of the truth of Goethe's primary phenomenon and the correctness of his whole theory of physical colors. Starting simply from the knowledge of color in the strictest sense, hence as a phenomenon in the eye, we have found that its external cause must be a diminished light, yet diminished in a definite way, which must have the characteristic of imparting just as much light to the color as it imparts darkness, σκιερόν, to the complement of that color. But this can happen infallibly, and in a way suitable to all cases, only by the cause of brightness in a given color being precisely the cause of the shade or darkness in its complement. For *conversa causa, convertitur effectus.*[7] Now this requirement is completely satisfied only by the partition of opacity inserted between light and darkness, because under opposite illumination it always causes two physiologically complementary colors. These colors turn out differently according to the degree of thickness and density of this opacity, but together they compose white, that is to say, the full activity of the retina. With the minimum thinness of the opacity, these colors will be yellow and violet; with increasing density, they will gradually change into orange and blue; and finally, with still greater density, they become red and green. These last, however, cannot be really demonstrated in this simple way, although the sky at sunrise and sunset occasionally gives us a feeble representation of it. When the opacity is complete, that is, when it becomes so dense as to be impervious to light, then, with light falling on it, white appears, and, with light placed behind it, darkness or black. – As a result of deriving Goethe's "primary phenomenon" from my theory, it no longer deserves to be called this. For it is not, as Goethe took it to be, something simply given and for-

7. ["With reversal of the cause, reversal of the effect." –*Trans.*]

ever withdrawn from all explanation; on the contrary, it is only the cause, required in consequence of my theory, for producing the effect and thus for halving the activity of the retina. The only primary phenomenon, in the proper sense, is that organic capacity of the retina to let its nervous activity appear in two qualitatively opposite halves, sometimes equal, sometimes unequal, and to throw them successively into relief. Here, of course, we must stop, because from this point – a point we often reach in physiology – we can see, at best, only final causes. Thus, we eventually have, through color, one more means of distinguishing and recognizing things.

From the derivation of Goethe's primary phenomenon given here, it follows also that the physical contrast must always correspond to, and agree with, the physiological. In the four colors, which the prismatic spectrum exhibits originally and in the simplest state, it fully corroborates what has been said, as can be readily seen from the sketch of this derivation given above. Thus the doubly dense cloudiness of a double subsidiary image produces on, the one side the blue band and, on the other side, the yellowish-red, thus two complements to the retina's full activity. The cloudiness that is half as dense gives in corresponding places the violet and yellow edges, which are also complementary. Thus the physical and physiological contrasts wholly correspond to one another. In just the same way, certain turbid solutions of quassia, lignum nephriticum, and the like give, in the case of transmitted light, that same yellow, which is the complementary color of blue and which they exhibit in the case of incident light. Even tobacco smoke appears a dull orange when blown toward the light and blue when blown towards the shady side. – As a result of all this, the physical contrast of yellow and blue put forward by Goethe holds good only in a general way, that is to say, only insofar as yellow and blue do not here signify two colors but two classes of colors. It is necessary to note this restriction. Now if Goethe goes still further and calls this physical contrast of yellow and blue a polar contrast, then I could agree with him only by means of an extremely farfetched interpretation, and I must differ from him. For, as my whole interpretation shows and reveals, only colors in the strictest sense have polar contrasts, that is to say, colors as affections of the retina, the polarization of which is the separation into qualitatively opposite activities. To maintain the polarity of light is equivalent to maintaining the partition of light. Since Goethe rejects the latter, but yet speaks of a polarity of colors independent of the eye, and explains color itself from the conflict of light with cloudiness or darkness, not tracing its origin any further, then this polarity of color could be nothing else but a polarity of this conflict. The inadmissibility of this assertion requires no further explanation. Every polarity must spring from a unity; it is this unity's disunion with itself, its separation into two qualitative opposites. But polarity can never, in any way, result from the chance encounter of two things of different origin, such as light and a dull or cloudy medium.

Finally, as regards chemical color, it is obviously a peculiar modification of the surface of bodies, a modification that is so fine we cannot possibly recognize and distinguish it but that alone makes itself known by the ability to produce this or that definite half of the eye's activity. For us this ability is still a *qualitas occulta*. But it is easy to see that so fine and delicate a modification of surface can be violently changed, even by trifling circumstances, and therefore cannot stand in any relation or connection with the inner and essential properties of the body. This extreme readiness of chemical colors to change goes so far that only an exceedingly small change, or one that cannot even be detected, in the properties of the body, in which the color is inherent, corresponds to a total change of color. Thus for example, the cinnabar obtained from the fusion of mercury and sulphur is black – just like a similar combination of lead with sulphur. Only after it has been sublimated does cinnabar assume the well-known fiery-red color, and yet it is not possible to demonstrate a chemical change in it. By merely warming it, red mercuric oxide becomes brownish black, and yellow basic nitrate of mercury becomes red. A well-known Chinese face powder arrives laid on little pieces of cardboard and is dark green, but when touched with the moistened finger it instantly is colored bright red. Even crabs turning red through boiling can be mentioned in this connection, as can the sudden change of many leaves from green to red at the first frost, and the turning red of apples on the side that receives the sun. One might ascribe this to a more powerful deoxidation of this side, in just the same way that some plants have the stem and the whole outline of the leaf in bright red but the parenchyma in green; also, in general, the diversity of colors in many petals of flowers and the many varieties of color of one kind, such as in tulips, carnations, mallows, dahlias, etc. In other cases, we can show that the chemical difference revealed by color is a very small one, for example, when tincture of litmus or violet extract change their color through the slightest trace of oxidation or alkalinization.

All this confirms, on the one hand, the predominatingly subjective nature of color resulting from my theory. This has always been felt, as is testified by the old proverb "*des goûts et des couleurs il ne faut disputer*"[8] and the proverb "*nimium non crede colori*,"[9] which has proved true. For this reason, color has well nigh become the symbol of deceitfulness and inconstancy, so that it has always been found hazardous for one to confine oneself to color. For this reason we have to be careful not to attach too much importance to colors in nature. On the other hand, the examples quoted tell us that the *eye is the most sensitive reagent* in the chemical sense, since it enables us to recognize instantaneously not only the most trifling change that can be demonstrated but even such changes of combination and composition that no other reagent can indicate. This incomparable sensitivity of the eye generally depends on the possibility of *chemical* colors, which in itself is still wholly unexplained. Through Goethe we have at last arrived at a correct insight into *physical* colors, despite the fact that Newton's well-advertised and false theory rendered this more difficult. The relation between physical and chemical colors is entirely similar to that between the magnetism produced by galvanic apparatus and to this extent intelligible from its immediate cause, and the magnetism fixed in steel and iron ores. The former furnishes a temporary magnetism that exists only by a complicated set of circumstances and ceases to exist as soon as they are abolished. The latter, on the contrary, is inherent in a body; it is unalterable and so far unexplained. It is bewitched, like an enchanted prince. Now the same holds true with the chemical color of a body. Thus tourmalines, in which a fleeting electricity can be produced merely by friction, furnish us with another comparison. For just as chemical colors merely require illumination to appear – in contrast to physical colors, which appear only by a combination of circumstances – so tourmalines merely require warming in order to reveal the electricity that at all times resides in them.

A general explanation of chemical colors appears to me to lie in the following. Light and heat are metamorphoses of each other. The sun's rays are cold so long as they illuminate; only when they impinge on a body impervious to light and cease to illuminate does their light change into heat. Thus,[10] by passing through a thin sheet of ice into an

8. ["One must not argue about tastes and colors." –*Trans.*]
9. ["Do not believe too much in color!" –*Trans.*]
10.* The experiment by Saussure is mentioned by Schelling in *Weltseele*, p. 38.

internally charred box, they raise the thermometer to a considerable degree without melting the sheet of ice. Even a lens frosted over with ice burns an object placed at its focal point without melting the ice. – This could never be if there were original and unalterable rays of heat, different from light rays, that, mixed with these, would be emitted by the sun, would as such pass through the ice, and thus act and inevitably melt it. (*A glass bell* placed over a plant produces a high degree of warmth because the light passes through instantaneously and is converted into warmth on the opaque ground. The glass, however, is not so readily permeable to this warmth as it is to light; it therefore accumulates under the glass bell and reaches a high degree.) On the contrary, heat is changed into light when stones are made red-hot, when glass is annealed, when metals are heated (even in irrespirable gasses), and when fluorspar is melted even with slight warming. The specially modified way in which an object, according to its state or condition, changes the light that falls on it into heat, is, for our eye, its chemical color. This color turns out to be darker the more readily and completely this process of change takes place; thus black bodies most easily become warm. This is all that we know about it. Yet we can understand from this how the different colors of the prismatic spectrum warm bodies in different ways. Even assuming the colors of the prismatic spectrum, we can also see how a merely physical color can produce a chemical color, for example chloride of silver being turned black by free, hence white, sunlight, if the chloride of silver remains exposed to it for a long time. Here the arising chemical color is, for our eye, the expression of the modified and enfeebled way in which the chloride of silver receives the light and converts it into heat, while the free and unchecked course of this process with white light is made manifest by the color turning black. – As heat and light are metamorphosis of each other, so is *electricity* another metamorphoses of heat, as proved by Seebeck's thermoelectricity, where bismuth and antimony, when soldered to one another, at once convert into *electricity* the heat communicated to them. Electricity is converted into light by the electric spark and by current flowing in a vacuum. It is converted into heat when its current is impeded in the electrode, which, when iron, becomes white-hot and fuses.

The correctness of the fractions I have discovered, according to which the retina's activity is qualitatively divided in the case of the six principal colors, is obvious, as I have already said, but it remains a matter of direct judgment and must be taken as self-evident, because it is difficult, if not impossible, to demonstrate. However, I will mention two ways in which, if need be, it might be possible to find a proof. Frequent attempts have been made to find the exact determination of the ratios in which the three principal chemical colors should be mixed, in pairs, in order to produce the color exactly midway between them. Lichtenberg,[11] Erxleben,[12] and Lambert,[13] in particular, have been busy trying to answer this question. But only from my theory do we get the definition of the real significance of the problem as well as a scientific, and not merely an empirical, solution of it. I must, however, make the preliminary observation that the pigments to be used for these experiments must have absolutely perfect colors. (1)They must be colors that divide the whole activity of the eye without leaving an undivided remainder; that is, colors that are accordingly free from all paleness or darkness foreign to their whole nature and that are extremely glaring and energetic. (2) They must be colors that are exactly $1/3$, $1/2$, and $3/4$ of the eye's activity, hence perfect blue, red, and yellow; in other words, the three basic chemical colors in their highest purity. Now if by using such colors we wish to make green, which is $1/2$ the full activity, from blue, which is $1/3$, and yellow, which is $3/4$, then the quantity of blue must be to the quantity of yellow inversely as the difference between $1/3$ and $1/2$ is to the difference between $3/4$ and $1/2$. For as much as the one given color lies nearer to the required color than the other given color, so much more of it must be taken, and insofar as the other given color lies further from the required color, so much less of it must be taken. Therefore three parts of blue and two of yellow give perfect green. They should be mixed as dry powders, so that the pigments do not act chemically on each other, and they should be mixed according to volume and not to weight. The rule given in this example applies to every mixture of this kind. Now the exact agreement of the result with the numerical ratios of the different halves – halves into which the retina's activity separates out in the three principal pairs of colors – would furnish the proof of their correctness. But, of course, the judgment on the correctness of the result, as well as on the perfection

11. Note to the essay "De affinitate colorum," in *Operis ineditis Tobiae Mayeri, cura Lichtenberg* [1775, Bd. 1, s. 93ff. –*Trans.*])

12. *Physikalische Bibliothek*, Bd. 1, st. 4, s 403ff.

13. *Beschreibung einer [mit dem Calauschen Wachse ausgemalten, –Trans.] Farbenpyramide*, Berlin 1772.

of the colors used for the mixture, is always left to perception and sensation. This can never be set aside when we speak of colors. – Another way of establishing the proof of the numerical fractions that we are considering would be as follows. Let us procure perfectly black and perfectly white sand and mix them in six proportions, each exactly corresponding, in darkness, to one of the six principal colors. The result must then be that the ratio of black to white sand in the case of each color corresponds to the numerical fraction I have assigned to that color. Thus, for example, for a gray corresponding, in darkness, to yellow, we would take three parts of white and one part of black sand; whereas a gray corresponding to violet would require a mixture of sands in exactly the opposite proportion; green and red, on the contrary, would require equal proportions of black and white. However the difficulty arises here of determining which gray corresponds in darkness to each color. This could be decided by our observing the color close to the gray through a prism in order to see what relation of brightness to darkness each bears to the other in refraction. If in this respect they are both alike, then the refraction cannot give any color phenomenon.

§14
Some Additions to Goethe's Theory on the Origin of Physical Colors

First of all I will quote here a few agreeable facts that help to corroborate Goethe's fundamental law of physical colors but that he himself did not notice.

If in a dark room we cause the electricity of a conductor to flow through a glass vacuum tube, this electric light appears as a very beautiful *violet*. Here, as with blue flames, the light itself is at the same time the cloudy medium. For there is no essential difference whether the illuminated dimness through which we look into dark casts into our eye its own or reflected light. But since this electric light here is extremely faint and feeble, it gives rise to violet, fully in accordance with Goethe's theory, instead of causing blue like even the feeblest flame, such as that of sulphur, alcohol, etc.

A common, everyday proof of Goethe's theory, overlooked by him, is that bottles filled with red wine or dark beer that have been lying in a cellar for a long time often undergo a considerable cloudiness of the glass due to a deposit on the inside. As a consequence, they then appear light blue when the light falls on them, and also after they are emptied when we hold something black behind them. With light that shines through them, on the contrary, they show the color of the liquid or, when empty, the color of the glass.

Even the color of blue eyes is not a chemical but merely a physical color occurring in accordance with Goethe's law. For, according to Magendie's detailed account of the anatomy of the eye (*Précis élémentaire de physiologie*, vol. 1., deuxième édition, pp. 60, 61), the lining at the back of the iris is covered with a black material that immediately shines through brown or black eyes. With blue eyes, however, the texture of the iris is whitish – hence cloudy – and the underlying black layer shines through to produce the blue of the eyes. ("*Dans les yeux bleus le tissu de l'iris est à peu près blanc; c'est la couche noire postérieure, qui paraît à peu près seule et détermine la couleur des yeux.*") This is confirmed by Helmholtz, "Ueber das Sehn des Menschen," page 8. – It is just the same with the blue color of veins, which is also only physical. It originates because the darkish venous blood sheds a faint light through the walls of the blood vessels.

But the recently discovered planet Neptune is proof of Goethe's law on a grand scale. That is to say, the astronomical observations made by Father Secchi at the observatory of the Collegium Romanum and communicated to the *Comptes Rendus* of the 22nd September 1856 contain the definitely expressed statement that this great planet is *nebulous* (*nébuleux*) *and its color is sea blue* (*couleur de mer bleuâtre*). Naturally, because we have here a cloudiness illuminated by the sun with a dark ground behind it.

The colored rings that appear when we firmly press together with our fingers two polished pieces of plate glass or even two polished convex glasses, I explain in the following way. Glass has a considerable elasticity, so with this strong compression the surface to some extent gives and is flattened. For a moment it loses its perfect smoothness and evenness, resulting in a gradually increasing cloudiness akin to that exhibited by dully- polished glass. We have here, therefore, a cloudy medium and the different degrees of its cloudiness, with partly incident and partly transmitted light, give rise to the colored rings. If we release the pressure, the elasticity at once restores the previous condition of the glass, and the rings disappear. Some spirit dabbed over a polished glass gives such colors, only not in rings but in lines. There is here a perfect analogy with soap bubbles that were the cause of Newton considering colored rings in the first place. The soapy water is a cloudy medium; on the soap bubble it flows downwards at one moment and at another moment spreads sideways or even in an upward direction. It offers to the light alternating and varying degrees of cloudiness, which are precisely the cause of those colored rings and their change.[1]

With almost all newly discovered truths, one subsequently finds that there previously existed a trace of them, that something very like them had been said, that, in fact, such truths had been positively expressed without being noticed. This is often because the person enunciating them had not recognized their value and had not grasped the importance of their consequences, and this prevented their being developed. In those cases one had, if not the plant, at any rate the seed.

Thus we find half of Goethe's basic law of physical colors, or half of his primary phenomenon, already expressed by Aristotle in his *Meteorologica*, vol. 3, page 4:

> Φαίνεται τὸ λαμπρὸν διὰ τοῦ μέλανος ἢ ἐν τῷ μέλανι (διαφέρει γὰρ οὐδέν) φοινικυῦν . . . ὁρᾶν δ' ἔξεστι τό γε τῶν χλωρῶν ξύλων πῦρ, ὡς ἐρυθρὰν ἔχει τήν φλόγα διὰ τὸ τῷ κ́απνῷ πολλῷ μεμῖχθαι τὸ πῦρ λαμπρὸν ὂν κ́αὶ λευκόν· καὶ δι' ἀχλύος καὶ καπνοῦ ὁ ἥλιος φαίνεται φοινικοῦς.

> (quodcunque fulgidum est, per atrum, aut in atro [nihil enim refert] puniceum apparet: videre enim licet ignem, e virentibus lignis conflatum, rubram flammam habere; porpterea quod ignis, suapte natura fulgidus albusque, multo fumo admixtus est: quin etiam sol ipse per caliginem et fumum puniceus apparet.)[2]

Stobaeus (*Eclogae physicae et ethicae*, vol. 1, p. 3l) repeats this in almost the same words as Aristotle's theory. The other half of Goethe's law has already been expounded by Leonardo da Vinci in his *Trattato della*

1.* In the *Revue des deux mondes*, 1 January 1858, Babinet says that the solar eclipse in March will be almost total and only one-tenth of the sun will remain; that the light of this passing through a narrow screen will cast on a screen not a circle, as on other occasions, but a thin, narrow lunar segment, similar to that of a new moon. This confirms Goethe's *theory of colors* because it proves that, as he teaches, it is not a pencil of rays passing through the *foramen exiguum* ["narrow slit," –*Trans.*] but a small *image of the sun*, which is then displaced by refraction.

2. ["Bright light shining through a dark medium or reflected in a dark surface (it makes no difference which) looks red. Thus one can see how the flames of a fire made of green wood are red, because the firelight that is bright and clear is mixed with a great deal of smoke; and the sun looks red when seen through mist or smoke"; p. 374a, –*Trans.*]

pittura, CLI. (See Brücke, *Ueber die Farben, welche trübe Medien im auffallenden und durchfallenden Lichte zeigen*, 1854, p. 10.) I cannot help observing that my theory of colors is a fortunate exception to this almost universal fate that has evoked the curse: "*pereant qui ante nos nostra dixerunt*!"[3] For, prior to 1816, never at any time did it occur to anyone to regard color, this phenomenon that is so objective, as the halved activity of the retina, and accordingly to assign to each individual color its *definite numerical fraction* – a fraction that, with another color, goes to make up unity, this unity then representing white or the full activity of the retina. And yet these fractions are so positively obvious that Professor Rosas, who would like to appropriate them, introduces them as absolutely self-evident in his *Handbuch der Augenheilkunde*, 1830, volume 1, Section 535 and also page 308. Hence I can say with Giordano Bruno:

> *Obductum tenuitque diu quod tempus avarum,*
> *Mi liceat densis promere de tenebris.*[4]

Since 1816 many, of course, have tried to smuggle them in as their own wares. They have made absolutely no mention of me, or only in such a casual way that no one suspects it.

Only on two points have I been compelled to differ from Goethe in my theory; namely, in regard to the true polarity of colors, as explained above, and in regard to the production of white from colors. Goethe has never forgiven me for the latter, yet he has never advanced any argument against it, either verbally or in writing.

But these two departures from Goethe will appear all the more honest and the outcome of purely objective reasons, as I am convinced of the merit and value of his work and deem it fully worthy of having as its author one of the greatest minds of all time. But even when it has such an origin, a newly created theory at the very moment of its birth can hardly ever be so perfect, without a miracle, that nothing remains for a successor either to add or to correct. Therefore, if there are errors indicated by me and possibly others in Goethe's work, this is of small significance compared with the truth of the whole, and this defect is completely removed by its great merit.

3. ["Down with those who have spoken our thoughts before us!" –*Trans.*]

4. ["And what avaricious time steadily concealed so long I bring forth – it was permitted me! – deep from the darkness." –*Trans.*]

This merit consists in having exposed and unmasked that strange mixture of self-deception and deliberate delusion, revered and believed in for two hundred years, and, at the same time, in furnishing a generally correct description of that part of nature that has taken into consideration:

> Μηδὲν ἁμαρτεῖν ἐστι ϑεῶν καὶ πάντα κατορϑοῦν·
> ᾿Εν βιοτῇ μοῖραν δ᾿ οὔτι φυγεῖν ἔπορον!.[5]

It is incumbent on us to acknowledge what has been accomplished, to accept it gratefully and with good sense, and then to the best of our ability improve it to the greatest possible extent.

Until now, of course, the opposite of this has occurred. Goethe's theory of color has met not merely a cold, but a positively unfavorable, reception. Indeed (*crediti posteri!*)[6] it fell flat right from the beginning, since it publicly suffered the unanimous condemnation of professionals from all sides and without proper opposition. On the authority of these people, the rest of the educated public, already predisposed by indolence and indifference, is glad to dispense with its own verification. Therefore even now, after forty-four years, it is content with things as they are. So this work of Goethe shares with many works of earlier ages, which are granted superior status by their subject and not by their treatment, the honor of having been put to one side almost untouched for many years after its appearance. And even during the present day, Newton's theory is spread abroad without interruption by all the professors and is now, as always, harped on in compendiums.

In order to understand this fate of Goethe's theory of colors, we must not disregard how great and pernicious is the influence exercised by the *will* [*Wille*] on all the sciences, indeed on all achievements of the mind, that is, by biases, and to speak more precisely, by bad and mean biases. In Germany, the fatherland of Goethe's scientific achievement, its fate is the least excusable. Eastlake, the painter and gallery inspector, furnished his countrymen, in 1840, with such an excellent translation of Goethe's theory of color that it is a perfect reproduction of the original and reads more easily; in fact, it is understood more easily than the original. We must see how Brewster behaves when reviewing it in the *Edinburgh Review*, that is to say, not unlike a tigress

5. ["Never to err and never to miss the mark are the business of the gods: to mortals it is not granted to escape their fate." –*Trans.*]

6. ["Believe in posterity!" –*Trans.*]

when someone rushes into her den to snatch away her cubs. Is this the tone of calm and certain conviction in the face of the errors of a great man? On the contrary, it is the tone of the intellectually bad conscience that feels with alarm that the opposite side is right, and is now resolved to defend, πὺξ καὶ λάξ[7] as a national treasure, the pseudo-science that is thoughtlessly accepted without investigation. By adhering to it, one has already been compromised. Now if Newton's color theory is accepted by the English as a national affair, then a good French translation of Goethe's work would be highly desirable; for we would then certainly hope to see justice done by the French learned world, which is neutral in this matter. Yet we see even them deeply compromised in this matter by the doctrines of ether vibrations, thermochrose, interference, and so on, all based entirely on the theory of homogeneous rays of light. Hence from their allegiance to Newton's theory of color there arise amusing and entertaining problems. For example, Biot relates with heartfelt approval in the *Journal des Savants*, April 1836, how Arago carried out very clever experiments in order to determine whether the seven homogenous light rays might not have an unequal velocity of propagation, so that from the variable fixed stars that are now nearer, now more distant, red, or possibly violet, light arrives first, and thus the star appears to assume different colors in succession. But, fortunately, he finally stated that this was not so. *Sancta simplicitas*![8] – Mr. Becquerel also does quite nicely in a *Mémoire présenté à l'académie des sciences*, le 13 juin 1842, in which he chants afresh the same old tune before the academy, as if it were something new:

> si on réfracte un faisceau [!] de rayons solaires à travers un prisme, on distingue *assez nettement* [here his conscience is knocking at the door] sept sortes de couleurs, qui sont: le rouge, l'orangé, le jaune, le vert, le bleu, l'indigo [this mixture of 3/4 black with 1/4 blue is supposed to be found in light!] et le violet.[9]

As Mr. Becquerel still has the effrontery to repeat this extract from

7. ["Tooth and nail." –*Trans.*]

8. ["Sacred simplicity." When he was burning at the stake, Johann Hus was alleged to have said this to a peasant who fed a piece of wood into the flames. –*Trans.*]

9. ["If we reflect a pencil of solar rays through a prism [of flint-glass and receive the oblong refracted image on a white card], we distinguish *clearly enough* . . . seven kinds of colors or seven parts of the image, each of which is colored with approximately the-same tint. These colors are red, orange, yellow, green, blue, indigo . . . and violet." –*Trans.*]

the Newtonian credo with such fearlessness and unconcern thirty-two years after the appearance of Goethe's color theory, we might feel tempted to declare to him, *assez nettement,* [10] "either your are blind or you are lying." Yet we would be doing him an injustice, for it is simply a case of Mr. Becquerel having more faith in Newton than in his own two eyes. This is the effect of the Newtonian superstition. – It is worthwhile mentioning specially the large two-volume compendium of physics (*Élémens de Physique*) by Pouillet that, by order of the government, is the foundation of public instruction in France. Here (Book 6, part I, chapter 3) we find the whole of Newton's revealed doctrine of color given on twenty large pages with certainty and boldness as if it were gospel, and with all Newton's tricks, together with their cautiousness and artifice. Whoever is intimately acquainted with the true state of affairs and with the connection between facts will read this chapter with great indignation, although at times this will be punctuated with laughter. For one will see how the false and absurd are imposed anew on the rising generation by completely silencing all refutation – a colossal *ignoratio elenchi*![11] – The most revolting thing is the care with which the minor details and incidents are quoted; they are calculated merely to deceive and are otherwise completely groundless; among them are even a few of later invention. This betrays the constant purpose of deception. For example, at Section 392, no. 3 (édition de Paris 1847) an experiment is described that is supposed to prove that white is produced by the combination of the seven so-called prismatic colors. A cardboard disk of one foot diameter is painted with *two circular black zones*, one around the circumference, the other around the center. Between the two zones are pasted paper strips tinted with the seven prismatic colors, each of which is frequently repeated, and running in the direction of the radii. The disk is now set spinning rapidly, and the color zone is supposed to appear *white*. Of the two *black zones*, however, not a syllable is given to account for them, nor could any account be honestly given, because they quite needlessly reduce the color zone that is alone relevant to the problem. So what is their point? – This is what Goethe would have said at once; in his absence I must now say it: in order that the contrast and the physiological aftereffect of black may

10. ["Clearly enough." –*Trans.*]
11. ["Irrelevant conclusion." –*Trans.*]

render the "base gray" produced, simply by this mixture of colors, so conspicuous that it can pass for white. Thus are the young students of France duped by such conjuring tricks, *in majorem Neutoni gloriam.*[12] For Goethe set the following piece to tune before the considerable improvement through the two black zones, which are a recent invention:

> To show Newtonian white to children
> Who bow at once to earnest pedagogues,
> There once appeared a teacher with the
> farce of the whirling wheel.
> On this was formed a circle of color.
> "Look at it closely with me! What do you
> see, my lad?" What do I see? Is it gray?
> "You don't see right! Do you think I'll
> allow this? White, you fool, white! Thus
> says Mollweide."
>
> [*Dem Weißmacher*]

This obstinate adherence to the Newtonian theory of colors and the wholly *objective* existence of color has had its revenge on physicists by leading them to a mechanical and clumsy color theory along the lines of Descartes or even of Democritus. According to this theory, color is supposed to depend on the variation in the vibrations of a certain ether, with which they are intimately acquainted, and of which they make bold and lavish use, but which is a wholly hypothetical, indeed a mythical and entirely unfounded, substance.[13] Even if ether existed, the fact that it might *possibly* have been indirectly the cause of a premature arrival of a comet, which is assumed on the strength of a calculation – from this fact, no one would admit it as a proof of the existence of ether. (Against Enke's explanation of the acceleration of his comet from the resistance of the ether, Bessel has declared and stated from the very beginning that one could specify a hundred caus es from which this acceleration could just as well be explained; cf. *Comptes rendus*, 6 December 1858, p. 893.) But now they confidently set to work on exact calculations of the imaginary lengths of the imaginary oscillations of an imaginary ether; for they are satisfied if only they have numbers, and thus the aforesaid lengths of oscillation are complacently calculated into millionths of a millimeter. In addition

12. ["For the greater glory of Newton." –*Trans.*]
13.* See *The World as Will and Representation*, 3rd ed., vol. 2, p. 358 et seq. [315-16, –*Trans.*].

we have here the amusing fact that they assign the *most rapid* oscillations to violet, the darkest and least effective of all the colors; on the other hand, they assign the least rapid oscillations to red, which affects our eye so vividly and which causes a commotion even among animals. But as I have already remarked, colors are for them mere names; they do not really perceive colors, but start with calculations, the element in which they feel at home.

Moreover, we have not to guard merely against the theory of these modern Newtonian chromotologists but will do well to look twice at their facts and experiments. There are, for instance, the Frauenhofer lines, about which so much fuss has been made, and about which it is assumed that they exist in light itself or are the interstices of the separate, extremely numerous, really homogeneous rays of light; thus they are even assumed to be differently constituted according to whether it is the light of the sun, Venus, Syrius, lightning, or a lamp. I have made repeated experiments with excellent instruments fully in accord with Pouillet's instructions without ever obtaining the linear. I had abolished it when the German version of Pouillet by J. Müller happened to come into my hands. This honest German tells us (2d ed., vol. 1, p. 416) what Pouillet discreetly suppresses, namely that the lines do not appear unless a second slit is introduced immediately in front of the prism. This confirmed my previous opinion that the only cause of these lines are the edges of the slit. For that reason I wish that someone who will not shun the difficulties and intricacies would prepare slits that are arched, or winding, or finely toothed (from brass and with screws like those in ordinary use). It is then highly probable that the Frauenhofer lines, to the scandal of the learned world, will betray their true origin by their shape – just as a child conceived in adultery betrays its father by its likeness to him. Indeed this is all the more probable as it squares with the experiment, mentioned by Pouillet (vol. 1, Section 365), of letting the light fall through a small, round hole onto a white surface. There are then supposed to be a number of concentric rings in the luminous circle that appears. These rings likewise failed to appear for me, and the honest Müller informs us (Vol. I, Section 218) that a second hole, introduced in front of the first, is required. In fact he adds that, if we use a fine slit instead of this hole, then parallel streaks appear instead of concentric rings. Then we have Frauenhofer lines! I cannot help expressing the wish that someday a good and unprejudiced head will, quite independently of Newton's theory and of the mythical oscillations of ether, take all the highly complicated chromatic experiments, collected mainly by French opticians and Frauenhofer, including the so-called polarization of light and interference, and endeavor to find out the true connection between all these phenomena. For the increase in intelligence has by no means kept pace with the increase in the number of facts; on the contrary, it lamentably lags behind. This is quite natural, because everyone is able to increase experience, especially by the accumulation and complication of conditions, but only a few can explain and interpret it. Generally speaking, physicists, especially in our day, have usually been concerned less with the *grounds* [*Gründe*] than with the *consequences* of natural forces. They are more concerned with their effects and consequently with their different applications, e.g., with the use of the force of elastic vapors for machines, steamships, and locomotives, or with the use of electromagnetism for telegraphs, achromatism for telescopes, and so on. In this way they gain the respect of ordinary people. Yet as far as the grounds are concerned, things are in a fair way and, for example, they are tarred with the same Newtonian brush, and, as little as they are in keeping with this, they must conform by hook or by crook.

If the spectrum comes from electric light, the Frauenhofer lines are supposed to be bright instead of black (see Pouillet). In a detailed account of them, "Sur la lumière électrique par Masson," in the *Comptes rendus de l'àcadémie des sciences*, 16 April 1855, it is stated, after accurate investigation, that the cause of these *rayes brillantes* are the incandescent metallic particles of the electrodes, in contact when the circuit is closed, which are torn adrift by the heat and pulled upwards by the electric current. If the electric spark is produced under water, they fail to appear.

On the *polarization of light* the *French* have nothing but nonsensical theories from the theories of undulation and homogeneous rays of light, together with calculations that are based on nothing. They are always in a hurry to measure and calculate; they always regard these as the main thing, and their battle cry is *le calcul! le calcul!* [14] But I say: *Où le calcul commence l' intelligence des phénomènes cesse.*[15] When a man has in his head mere numbers and signs, he cannot obtain an inkling of causal connections. How much and how big are of importance for *practical* purposes; but in theory the chief thing that comes first is the

14. ["Arithmetic! Arithmetic!" –*Trans.*]
15. ["Where arithmetic begins, understanding of the phenomena ceases." –*Trans.*]

What. Reaching this, we make sufficient progress with a rough estimation concerning the how much and the how big.

Goethe was too old when these phenomena were discovered – he was beginning to talk foolishly.

I explain the matter generally as follows. The reflection of light at an angle of 35 degrees actually splits up the light into two different components, of which the reflected part displays special properties. But all of these revert to the fact that this light, now deprived of an integral component, appears weak and feeble but thereby shows a marked tendency to produce physical colors; for every physical color originates from a particular dimness or enfeeblement of light. Therefore, it displays this specific enfeeblement first of all in its furnishing only one of the two images of Iceland spar; thus the other image arose in consequence of the other component of light, now eliminated. Then it cannot completely fill the rapidly cooled glass cube, yet it is not uniformly diffused, but is concentrated. In this way it illuminates some places and leaves others blank; these appear black and in certain positions form a cross, but properly speaking, they show two black bands that are flexible. As we turn the cube around, these bands now pass through it in all directions in the form of waves; now they form a black border and come together in the middle like an X, thus exhibiting a cross only when the cube has its side turned horizontally to the eye. Yet in order to see all this clearly, a *parallelepiped*, and the cube proper, is the most suitable glass body. By rotation, the four yellow spots in the angle of the cross can also be spread into stripes on the edge. On the whole they are evidence of the great tendency of this light, deprived of an integral component, to produce physical colors, of which yellow, as is well known, is the one most easily formed. The aforesaid tendency shows itself in all sorts of phenomena. Mica or spar laminae, placed on the cube or on each other, display all kinds of colors. The production of Newton's rings by plate glass or lenses always normally requires a certain pressure; they arise in polarized light with the greatest of ease. In particular, two polished sheets of rock crystal produce them in great beauty and marvelous uniformity without any other pressure other than their own weight.

The most marvelous sight of polarized light is, of course, that provided by a piece of Iceland spar clamped between two sheets of tourmaline. It displays a black or white cross, according to its position, and this cross is surrounded by an aureole of Newtonian rings. It seems certain that the Iceland spar also polarizes the light (produces like reflection in the angle of 35 degrees). It must therefore be possible to derive this marvel from the above principles. –

The grave injustice, which Goethe must have suffered in regard to his theory of color has many different causes, and to enumerate them all would be as inconsiderate as it would be unpleasant. We can, however, express one of them in the words of Horace:

> turpe putant, [parere minoribus et] quae
> imberbi didicere, senes perdenda fateri.[16]

The same fate, however, has befallen every significant discovery as long as it was new, as is testified by the history of all the sciences. It is something which will not surprise the few who have the insight to see "that the excellent is rarely found and more rarely appreciated,"[17] and "that the absurd really engrosses the world."[18] However, the day of justice for Goethe's color theory will not fail to come, and then a saying of Helvetius will once more be confirmed, namely that, "*le mérite est comme la poudre: son explosion est d'autant plus forte, qu'elle est plus comprimée* (*De l'esprit*, disc. 2, ch. 10),[19] and then the oft repeated drama in the history of literature will be played afresh and brought to an end.

But the descendant, the one descendant out of millions, who will be conscious of his power to bring forth something original, new, extraordinary in art or science, and who therefore will likely meet some old fashion in art, though in science will certainly meet some old delusion in opposition, will someday become familiar with the history of Goethe's theory of colors before he passes his work on to his contemporaries. From the *Optics*, which will then rest in the libraries only as material for literary history, he will become acquainted with the Newtonian ghost that has long since ceased to haunt any head. Afterwards, he will read Goethe's color theory for himself, the main points of which will have been briefly and concisely impressed on him in school. Finally, he will also read the documents of the reception of Goethe's work, as much as the worms have left behind and his equanimity endures. Then he will compare the downright deceit, the

16. ["They hold it a shame to yield to their juniors, and to confess in their old age that what they learned in beardless youth should be destroyed." –*Trans.*]

17. [Goethe, *Wilhelm Meisters Lehrjahre*. –*Trans.*]

18. [Goethe, *Dichtung und Wahrheit*. –*Trans.*]

19. ["Merit is like powder: the more it is confined, the stronger its explosion." –*Trans.*]

conjuring-trick experiments of Newton's *Optics* with the so simple, so easily comprehensible, so unmistakable truths that Goethe enunciated. At last, he will bear in mind that Goethe came forward with his work at a time when the well-deserved laurel wreath crowned his worthy head and he received, at least from the most noble of his time, fame and admiration that still matched to some extent his deserts and greatness of spirit, at a time, therefore, when he was certain to attract universal attention. – And then he will see how little, how even none of this, was able to do anything against that way of thinking which is now once more characteristic of the human race in general. After this observation, he will not draw back his hands; rather, completing his labor, because this work is the flower of his life that will bear fruit, he will pass it on, but knowing to whom, and ready.